Fasting for Health

Reset your Body Through Intermittent Fasting

Improve Health and Lose Weight

Anne Marie Houston

Table of Contents

Introduction

In the whirlwind of a dynamic corporate career, endless deadlines loomed overhead, and those global teams demanded my constant dedication and attention. I felt uncomfortable because of something that I didn't recognize happening beneath the day-to-day stress. I was facing an even greater challenge: a personal issue that affected my body in its entirety. I'm Anne Marie and much like you, my journey through the fast-moving corporate landscape left me not just with frequent flyer miles but also with excess weight and health issues.

In the pursuit of professional goals, my well-being took a backseat. This realization propelled me onto a transformative journey—one that unearthed the potency of diverse health initiatives. What unfolded was not just a revelation of various health options but a personalized exploration of what worked for my lifestyle.

Welcome to *Fasting for Health,* where I share not only factual insights but a narrative woven with personal experiences. I don't claim expertise; instead, I offer guidance gained from living through the remarkable transformation that intermittent fasting can bring. Recognition is not the goal; your well-being is the focal point of these pages.

So, what's this journey about? It's a reset achieved through intermittent fasting—a potent yet practical tool to enhance your physical and mental well-being. This isn't about deprivation; it's a strategic embrace of health, allowing you to relish food while reaping its benefits.

What Is Intermittent Fasting?

Before we delve deeper, let's understand the essence of intermittent fasting. It's not just a diet; it's a rhythm of eating. We'll explore various fasting options, unraveling the science behind them and providing you with a roadmap for your own fasting journey.

Fasting: A Historical Perspective

Briefly, let's glance back in time. Fasting isn't a trendy phenomenon; its roots trace back through history. This contextual glimpse sets the stage for our contemporary exploration, providing perspective without dwelling too long on the past.

So, why are we embarking on this journey together? The objectives are clear:

- This book aims to kindle inspiration within you and empower you to adopt a fasting lifestyle. It's not about deprivation or starving; it's about finding a balance that enhances both your physical and mental well-being.

- Equip yourself with the tools to navigate the fasting process, overcome challenges, and set achievable goals.

- Discover the myriad benefits of intermittent fasting, addressing a spectrum of health concerns. We'll also integrate exercise into this holistic approach to well-being.

In a world inundated with quick fixes and viral trends, *Fasting for Health* distinguishes itself by relying on facts and research rather than fads and TikTok hints. This book isn't a compilation of fleeting advice; it's grounded in substantiated information. The approach within is deliberate—no room for shortcuts or unverified claims. As you embark on this journey, rest assured that every piece of guidance is backed by reliable research, making this book a steadfast companion in your pursuit of health.

Chapter 1:

Understanding Intermittent

Fasting

The best of all medicines is resting and fasting. –Benjamin Franklin

Fasting isn't a word that's loved by many. Just the thought of skipping meals or leaving out a few tasty treats on the plate can bring about some frustration or moodiness. But, and this is a big but, fasting is more than the difficult act of depriving oneself of food. Just as the wise Benjamin Franklin said, it is a form of medicine. He recognized the healing potential embedded in two simple acts: resting and fasting. So, let's begin by unraveling layers of this wisdom and understanding how it sets the stage for our exploration of intermittent fasting.

The Essence of Rest and Fasting

Resting

In the world of fasting, you may wonder just what exactly rest has to do here. However, the importance of rest cannot be overlooked, as it is a foundational pillar for your overall health and well-being. Quality rest will play a vital role in supporting your body's natural healing processes, contributing to the repair and regeneration of tissues, and helping to maintain optimal immune function.

Sleep is intricately linked to your hormonal balance. Any disruption in your sleeping patterns will lead to imbalances in certain hormone levels, like insulin and cortisol, which are all very important when it comes to regulating your metabolism and energy levels. By prioritizing sufficient rest while practicing intermittent fasting, you will enhance the efficacy of your fasting periods, which promotes a synergistic relationship between rest and fasting for improved metabolic health (Fletcher, 2019).

Moreover, rest serves as a powerful aide for navigating the adjustments and challenges associated with intermittent fasting. Keep in mind that during periods of fasting, your body is going to undergo various metabolic shifts, and rest will become a supportive mechanism to not only manage stress levels but reduce inflammation as well. Quality sleep is going to aid in the mitigation of the potential negative effects of fasting, like irritability and fatigue. And this is achieved by fostering a sense of calm and promoting mental resilience. Integrating restful practices like mindfulness and relaxation techniques into your fasting routine will further enhance the holistic approach to intermittent fasting. This is going to create a harmonious balance between healing and rejuvenation, enhancing overall health benefits.

Fasting

Now, moving on to intermittent fasting, this is going to open the door to a transformative approach to health and well-being. Remember that fasting isn't a new method to obtain health or lose weight. It is an ancient practice with deep roots in various cultures and religions. It has gained renewed attention for its potential benefits in the realm of the modern world, but at its core, fasting involves cycling between periods of eating and fasting, presenting a departure from the traditional dietary patterns that we have come to observe. Keep in mind that this approach will not only challenge conventional notions about meal timing but also tap into the body's inherent ability to adapt and optimize its functions.

Now, those knowledgeable in the fields of biology and science would find this questionable. Wouldn't this method cause you to gain more weight than lose it? After all, if your body thinks it is starving, it will save every bit of sugar you take in and convert it into fat, which will cause more weight gain. Well, let's break down how the body works—from ingestion to the breakdown and usage of fat—to explain this.

When you consume food, your body breaks down fats and sugars to absorb essential nutrients for energy. Subsequently, these nutrients are utilized for various purposes, such as boosting the immune system and building muscle fibers. Any excess or unnecessary components are eliminated from the body. Delving further into the nutritional aspect, the types of nutrients present in a meal, such as vitamins, minerals, salt, sugar, fats, and water, depend on its quality. Nutrient-rich meals contribute positively, while processed or "dead" foods lack nutritional value.

The body selectively absorbs and utilizes nutritious elements from the ingested food. Excess energy from meals high in sugar and fats is converted into fat and stored in specific body areas (*Building, Burning, and Storing: How Cells Use Food*, n.d.). Consuming more calories than your body requires leads to fat accumulation, resulting in weight gain (Villines, 2021).

To prevent weight gain, it is essential to eat at the right intervals. This allows your body to efficiently utilize the energy intake, preventing the storage of surplus calories as fat.

Now, let's move on to a misconception where people believe that any type of fasting method is the same thing. However, the downside of fasting using an unapproved method or doing something without doing any research could lead to many issues down the line. For example, the issue of not eating enough for your body to use and limiting the nutrients that your body needs to survive will cause major havoc on your system. This will result in issues that will cause more harm than good and will decrease your motivation to try again with fasting.

Employing a researched system compels your body to efficiently utilize the sugar and fat intake, a process enhanced by intermittent fasting that minimizes the likelihood of overeating. The mechanism behind this involves the conversion of stored sugar and starch into fat. When your body lacks the necessary daily nutritional value, it taps into these stored fats, converting them into glucose to elevate blood sugar levels, thereby providing the energy needed for day-to-day functions.

In essence, intermittent fasting promotes digestion, absorption, and utilization of nutrients while also facilitating the burning of excess or stored fat in the body. It's crucial to recognize that intermittent fasting extends beyond mere abstinence from eating; it constitutes a comprehensive lifestyle choice encompassing mindful nutrition, strategic meal timing, and acknowledging the profound impact of rest on metabolic balance.

As we delve into the specifics of intermittent fasting, it's essential to grasp that there are four distinct types, each offering a unique rhythm of potential health benefits.

And yes, when it comes to intermittent fasting, we are going to encounter a spectrum of approaches that offer a unique rhythm to the rest and fasting equation. Let's dissect these methods and explore their nuances, benefits, and considerations.

16/8 Method

Try to imagine yourself living a life where you aren't fixated on *what* you are going to eat but rather on *when* you are eating. This is the essence of the 16/8 method. It is based on a time-restricted eating window that gives your digestive system a schedule to work with. Now, it may sound a little difficult. How exactly are you going to eat for only eight hours a day and restrict eating for the rest of the 16 that's left? Well, look on the bright side. As you change your lifestyle and spend those 16 not-difficult but glorious hours in your fasting mode, your body taps into its fat stores for energy. Then, the curtain rises on the eight-hour eating window, where you will indulge in a few of your favorite meals. Think of it as a culinary concert for your metabolism.

This method's primary advantages go beyond the simple pastime of watching clocks. Your body's natural rhythm will encourage enhanced insulin sensitivity, fat burning, and better digestion. Studies even suggest that this approach might be your key to losing weight without requiring you to have backstage passes to the gym (*Intermittent Fasting: What Is It, and How Does It Work?*, 2023). This does not, however, relieve you of the necessity to work out every day.

Sarah was a graphic designer that I knew personally. During her earlier years, she was fun to be around and energetic, but as time went on, things changed. Because of the responsibilities in both her personal and professional life, she started to feel moody, lethargic, and lacking in energy. Upon learning about intermittent fasting, she decided to replace her midnight munchies with a full 16-hour window for fasting. She gradually became more energetic during the day and developed an unexpectedly fresh appreciation for her breakfast. The fasting method truly helped her come back to her usual chirpy self.

If the aforementioned advantages are not enough to catch your interest, this method has also revolutionized metabolic health in another way. By engaging in 16/8 method practice, you will allow your body to go into a transformational state. Your old cells are removed here to create space for your brand-new, shiny ones. Consider it a kind of cell-cleaning spring cleaning.

Let us take a look at some doable strategies you could use to integrate the 16/8 method into your everyday schedule.

Getting Practical

- Eat dinner early in the evening, around 7:00 p.m., to start your fasting symphony. This prepares the audience for the magic of fasting that comes next.

- On the day of the fast, break your fast at 11:00 a.m. Give your body permission to accept nutrition and begin the metabolic dance of the day.

- Consistency is paramount in the magnificent spectacle of intermittent fasting. Although this is a suggested rhythm, modify it to fit your way of life. Your rhythm should be reflected in the dance between eating and fasting. At first, it might seem difficult, but keep in mind that discipline is what turns difficulty into success.

- Do not be alarmed if the rhythm seems strange to you. If following the schedule starts to feel like work, give your stomach a little break. Eat a little piece of fruit when you are hungry; you could have a half-banana or a handful of grapes. Then, continue going longer between meals until you arrive at the appointed times with grace.

- Take deliberate steps to guide your routine.

- As you become skilled at intermittent fasting, acknowledge and celebrate each accomplishment. Savor the minute adjustments, the energy boosts, and the triumphs over cravings. Your health is like a symphony that you are conducting, and each note of discipline paves you one step closer to the encore of success.

Now, if you are thinking about using this approach, try to picture yourself as providing your digestive system with a much-needed vacation and your body with an opportunity to re-establish harmony with the natural rhythms that dictate its operations. But really, do not take my word for it; instead, as you set out on this incredible 16/8 adventure, let your body be the judge.

Now, let us move on to a different fasting strategy from the buffet that is more unusual and more alluring. Let's spice things up with a different kind of diet.

The 5:2 Diet

So here's where the dynamic duo of feasting and fasting comes into play. I want you to hold on to your seat before we go any further because this diet is going to turn your regular eating habits into a culinary roller coaster. You might be wondering what's so good about this one because it seems strange to get so excited about something that will only slightly lessen your enjoyment of life. And if this is your first time taking this route, it might sound intimidating. But worry not. Let's answer all the questions you might have.

With this method, you will have five days of unrestricted feasting, and you get to enjoy your favorite meals without a care in the world. And then the plot thickens. From there, you will have to sacrifice two days of the week for calorie restriction, giving your metabolism a gentle nudge. Think of it as a weekend getaway for your digestive system. So, what exactly are the benefits? After all, it doesn't sound very fasting-like. Well, this dieting plan isn't just some numerical jigsaw; it's more of a metabolic masterpiece. Those two days that you set aside for your calorie restriction might seem like a challenge, but with research having gone into the system, we have found out that it could be your ticket to improved insulin sensitivity, brain function, and even a boost in longevity (*What Is the 5:2 Diet?*, n.d.).

To master the 5:2 diet, you will need to have balance. On the days when you get to feast, try to relish in the joy of culinary exploration. On your fasting days, opt for nutrient-dense foods to keep your body fueled and satisfied.

I once had a friend named Tom, who was an IT guru and spent most of his time in front of the screen. Because of this, he was eating unhealthy food and putting on a lot of weight. He wasn't enjoying his meals; he didn't feel satiated after eating. Looking back, he always had a packet of chips in front of him. When we both started our journeys into intermittent fasting, Tom had a connection with this dieting method. He transformed his weekend pizza binges into a structured 5:2 diet plan, and the result was that he wasn't just slimmer on the waistline; he also had a newfound appreciation for the art of moderation. He practiced mindful eating and was fuller for longer. He began to enjoy his meals.

If I had to talk about what sets the 5:2 diet apart, it would be its delightful flexibility. It invites you to dance between indulgence and restraint rather than requiring a drastic overhaul of your eating regimen. Intermittent calorie restriction has been the subject of much research, which promises a myriad of miraculous benefits ranging from improving metabolic health to triggering cellular repair processes (Schübel et al., 2016).

Now, let's map out your adventure in this culinary ballet. Consider it your self-help guide to embracing the 5:2 diet:

- Start by familiarizing yourself with the 5:2 diet's rhythm. Recognize that it is a moderate dance rather than a revolution in cuisine. Allow the health benefits and science underlying intermittent fasting to create a calming soundtrack.

- Make a weekly schedule that alternates between feast and fast days. On feast days, indulge in the flavors guilt-free and take in the nutrient symphony. Accept the challenge of fasting days like you would a dance partner, giving your body a chance to rest and recover.

- You will inevitably have moments of hunger, cravings, and uncertainty about the next steps. You will also inevitably experience surprises. Do not be afraid! This is normal. Keep a journal to record your emotions, and adjust the tempo as needed. For some comfort and support, get in touch with a reliable friend you may have told about the fast. If you find it extremely difficult, you can try what I did earlier and try eating some fruit or nuts and gradually extend the times that you do not eat. This will eventually help you get the hang of it.

- As you waltz through your 5:2 diet journey, celebrate the wins. Notice the subtle changes in energy, mood, and perhaps even in the way your favorite jeans fit. Revel in the fact that you're orchestrating a masterpiece—your own health and well-being.

So, dear reader, let the 5:2 diet be your culinary symphony, a masterpiece composed with every mindful bite and intentional fast. In this gastronomic ballet, you are both the conductor and the soloist, creating a harmonious tune that resonates with health and vitality. Onward to the feast!

Still skeptical? Imagine that implementing a 5:2 diet is similar to creating a harmonious blend of eating and fasting that keeps your metabolism bouncing. Well, I only urge you to hang on to your cooking skills—we have more delectable surprises in store for you at our fasting feast. Next on the menu is the eat-stop-eat method. Are you ready to unfold a 24-hour fasting fiesta?

The Eat-Stop-Eat Extravaganza

Let us enter the eat-stop-eat festival, where a full-day fasting carnival with the promise of an exhilarating metabolic experience will be the main attraction!

Imagine flipping the switch for a full day of fasting, perhaps twice a week, without stopping. That is the core of the eat-stop-eat approach, which upends your perception of meals and snacks and leaves your body in a state of severe maintenance.

One pro-tip to ensure that your body can keep up with fasting days is to stay well-hydrated to support your body through the challenge. Not only are water and herbal teas acceptable, but they also make great fasting companions during the day. During the fasting phase, these drinks can help ward off hunger and keep your energy levels stable.

When it is time to break your fast, make the most of it. Choose meals that are high in nutrients and offer a well-balanced combination of carbohydrates, healthy fats, and proteins. This deliberate approach maximizes the post-fast recovery phase while satisfying your hunger and making sure your body gets the vital nutrients it needs.

Let me introduce you to Alex, a fitness enthusiast whose resolve to maintain her physical appearance clashed with her busy schedule. Her energy levels declined, leaving her exhausted and mentally disoriented. This was caused by her erratic eating habits, frequent snacking, and consumption of processed foods. In an attempt to make a change, Alex made the decision to investigate the fascinating world of eat-stop-eat and give intermittent fasting a try. Everything changed after those 24-hour fasts, which began as an endurance test. The results were astounding: greater energy and an unexpectedly sharp mind renewed her workouts and had a profound impact on all facets of her life. Through this transformative event, Alex was able to get over her fatigue and find newfound energy, which gave her the strength and courage to take on challenges head-on. The remarkable results of eat-stop-eat are demonstrated by Alex's story, which alters not only physical health but also one's entire way of life and supports the notion that true wellness extends beyond the gym and into everyday life.

Remember that this is a complete metabolic symphony, not just another diet trick. When you embrace the longer fasting window of eat-stop-eat, your body will begin a dance known as autophagy—a cellular purification that leaves your interior architecture shining. Think of it as your body's detox adventure, giving your digestive system a well-earned vacation and an opportunity to concentrate on internal self-care. Now, let us examine a straightforward step-by-step guide that demonstrates how to effectively integrate this diet into your daily routine and eating patterns.

How to Carry It Out

- Recognize that the fundamental tenet of eat-stop-eat is to fast continuously for 24 hours once or twice a week. This entails consuming no calories for the entire day.

- Decide which days of the week you will add the 24-hour fast to your schedule. Once a week is the suggested starting point, and if comfortable, two times a week. Pick days that fit your lifestyle after taking your schedule into consideration.

- Give your fast a defined start and finish time. For example, you may choose to begin your fast at 7:00 p.m. after supper and end it at 7:00 p.m. the next day. Your fasting window will have a simple structure thanks to this.

- Make staying hydrated your top priority when fasting. A lot of water, herbal teas, and black coffee should be consumed. Consuming enough water during a fast can help reduce hunger and aid the body's healing process.

- Choose meals that are high in nutrients when you break your fast. After the fasting period, replenish your body with a balanced intake of protein, healthy fats, and carbohydrates.

Rich in nutrients, foods aid in the rejuvenation that occurs after the fast.

- Pay attention to your body throughout the fasting period. If you experience significant hunger or discomfort, consider easing into the practice with a small piece of fruit. Gradually extend the periods without food as your body adjusts.

- Consistency is key to seeing the benefits of eat-stop-eat. Stick to your chosen fasting days and times as much as possible. Building a consistent routine enhances the metabolic and health benefits associated with intermittent fasting.

- As you incorporate eat-stop-eat into your routine, celebrate the small victories. Notice changes in energy levels, mood, and overall well-being. Acknowledge your commitment to this fasting practice and its positive impact on your health.

Never forget how important it is to pay attention to your body and modify your strategy as necessary. Before making big dietary or fasting changes, speak with a healthcare provider, particularly if you have any pre-existing medical conditions.

Now, it's time to get ready for the magnetic allure of alternate-day fasting. Here, the fasting rhythm takes center stage in a one-of-a-kind groove. So, fasten your seatbelts and prepare for the next chapter of this fasting adventure; after all, the journey continues with a rhythmic twist!

Unlocking the Beat of Alternate-Day Fasting

The unique fasting method known as alternate-day fasting (ADF) upends customary meal schedules. The idea is straightforward but effective: alternate days of unlimited eating with complete fasts. This dance is rhythmic and requires your body to adjust to a varying pace that alternates between indulgence and restraint.

The possible health benefits of ADF make a beautiful melody. Studies indicate that it might help with weight loss, enhance cardiovascular health, and possibly lengthen life. Its sporadic challenge to your body's metabolism keeps it flexible and encourages the creative use of energy (Gupta, 2023).

The special selling point of ADF is its ability to trigger metabolic switching, which facilitates your body's effortless transition between burning fat and carbohydrates for energy. This adaptability is thought to be essential for improving resilience and metabolic health.

Allow me to introduce you to Emily, a graphic designer whose life was completely changed by ADF. Having trouble controlling her weight and energy levels, she accepted ADF as a possible remedy. On the fast, Emily lost extra weight and gained increased energy, mental clarity, and general well-being by being consistent and taking a thoughtful approach to her fasting days. ADF evolved from a food preference to a routine that improved her quality of life on a daily basis.

Detailed Instructions

- Consider your preferences, lifestyle, and health objectives before you jump in. Recognize the beat that complements your schedule and goals.

- To make sure that ADF is appropriate for your particular set of health needs and conditions, get advice from a medical professional.

- Choose the days you will fast. To stay hydrated on fasting days, drink lots of water, herbal teas, and black coffee.

- Eat a nutrient-dense, well-balanced diet on non-fasting days. Choose a balance of carbohydrates, healthy fats, and proteins.

- Observe the cues your body is sending you. If the rhythm seems too difficult at first, think about extending the fasting periods gradually to ease yourself into it.

- Just like Emily, adjust your strategy to meet your needs. Adapt the fasting schedule to your energy needs and way of life.

- Keep up a regular ADF schedule. Regular practice often leads to benefits.

Remember that the goal of this fasting journey is to discover a rhythm that improves your health and blends in perfectly with the overall melody of your life.

As we come to the end of our investigation into various fasting techniques, keep in mind that there is no one-size-fits-all strategy and that there is a wide variety of options. The key is to integrate any new health regimen you choose—be it the 16/8 method, the 5:2 diet, eat-stop-eat, or ADF—into your life in a way that is sustainable and pleasurable.

It is time to investigate the available options and suggestions to learn more about the special advantages of intermittent fasting.

Health Benefits of Intermittent Fasting

When it comes to health and well-being, intermittent fasting is a fascinating pattern that has significant advantages over traditional diets. Discovering the complex mechanisms at work as we explore this chapter will help you understand how intermittent fasting can promote weight loss, improve cognitive function and cardiovascular health, and even act as a preventative measure against aging and some diseases. Come explore with us the amazing world of metabolic miracles, cellular regeneration, and the health symphony created by intermittent fasting.

Wonder Weight Loss

Starting an intermittent fast sets off a series of metabolic adjustments that result in impressive weight loss. Fasting results in the following (Gunnars, 2021):

- The body's main energy store, glycogen, is depleted during the fasting phase. The body changes its metabolism in search of other fuel sources as a result of this depletion.

- When the body's supply of glycogen is depleted, it switches over smoothly to burning fat for energy, a metabolic state called ketosis. This change initiates the breakdown of fat cells to produce energy, a process known as lipolysis.

- The body breaks down fat cells in a methodical manner during lipolysis, which releases energy for different physiological processes. This process serves as the body's fuel during fasting and is the main cause of significant weight loss.

- Frequent periods of fasting serve as a training ground for the body to effectively use fat reserves as its main energy source. This adaptation plays a major role in the body's gradual weight loss and transformation into a toned, leaner shape.

- Regular intermittent fasting becomes a sculpting technique that shapes the body into a more elegant and slender form, going beyond simple weight loss. This process is a well-balanced combination of metabolic efficiency and fat utilization.

Weight loss through intermittent fasting is a life-changing experience that rewrites the rules about how the body and its energy sources interact. It is not just a band-aid solution. A lean, healthy body is something that can be sustained through the metabolic dance that fasting orchestrates.

Insulin Sensitivity Boost

A key factor in controlling blood sugar and improving insulin sensitivity is intermittent fasting, especially for prolonged periods of time. Let's take a closer look at the benefits:

- Intermittent fasting causes a reduction in blood glucose levels. This deliberate reduction creates the conditions for a series of positive metabolic effects.

- During fasting, the pancreas adjusts by producing less insulin in response to lower blood glucose levels. Better insulin sensitivity is a result of a fundamental change brought about by this measured response.

- Intermittent fasting actively reduces insulin resistance by releasing less insulin. This decrease in resistance enhances the body's capacity to regulate blood sugar by making cells more sensitive to insulin.

- Intermittent fasting results in increased insulin sensitivity, which protects against insulin-related health issues. One benefit of this is a decreased chance of type 2 diabetes and other metabolic diseases linked to insulin insufficiency.

- The promotion of stable blood sugar levels is the ultimate outcome of enhanced insulin sensitivity. Because they are now more adept at absorbing glucose, cells support a stable and balanced blood sugar environment.

Beyond diet fads, adopting intermittent fasting as a way of life becomes a deliberate strategy to support metabolic balance. Insulin sensitivity regulation establishes the foundation for a strong and stable physiological state in addition to offering protection against health risks.

Cellular Cleanup Crew (Autophagy)

There is no other process like the miracle of autophagy during intermittent fasting for cellular renewal.

- When you fast, your body goes into a state of meticulous cleaning that removes damaged proteins from your body. This cellular cleanup makes sure that broken parts are taken out quickly.

- Do note that autophagy is about optimizing cell function, not just tidying up. Cells can function at their best when damaged components are eliminated, which promotes general physiological health.

- Cell longevity is greatly impacted by autophagy's preventive function against the buildup of malfunctioning cellular components. It prolongs the life of your cells, much like a rejuvenating spa treatment.

- Your cellular landscape transforms in a revitalizing way when you fast intermittently, as autophagy facilitates cellular renewal and purging, which fosters an environment that supports cell viability and a feeling of youth.

- Also, autophagy orchestrates cellular cleanup that is not limited to a specific area of your body; it permeates your entire system and supports overall wellness. The restored cells support enhanced immunological response, organ function, and general physiological robustness.

Including intermittent fasting in your routine turns it from just a diet decision to a plan to mobilize your body's cellular cleanup team and keep your internal systems operating at peak performance. I think that the secret to extending life expectancy and cultivating an environment of internal health is autophagy's magic.

Enhanced Cognition

Intermittent fasting triggers the release of a crucial protein essential for optimal brain function, acting as a catalyst for enhanced cognition. This protein, known as brain-derived neurotrophic factor (BDNF), is released during fasting, initiating a series of positive neurological effects. BDNF plays a pivotal role in supporting the growth and maintenance of neurons, functioning as a growth factor. Additionally, it enhances brain flexibility by optimizing and adapting neuronal connections for more efficient cognitive processes.

The brain processes information more efficiently as a result of the increased synaptic plasticity. From there, a cognitive boost occurs, everyday tasks become clearer, and your thinking and memory sharpen.

Heart Health Superstar

Including periods of fasting in your routine helps you achieve mental and cognitive mastery in addition to supporting your physical health (Naous et al., 2023).

- Fasting intermittently reduces inflammatory markers, which in turn reduces chronic inflammation, a major contributing factor to heart disease.

- By reducing oxidative stress, fasting strengthens antioxidant defenses that protect cells from harm.

- Intermittent fasting helps to regulate blood pressure by addressing inflammation and oxidative stress, which lowers the risk of hypertension-related problems.

- The lipid profiles are affected by intermittent fasting, which encourages efficient cholesterol utilization and strengthens the cardiovascular system.

- Because of its combined effects on blood pressure, lipid profiles, inflammation, and oxidative stress, intermittent fasting is positioned as a heart-healthy habit that reduces the risk of cardiovascular diseases.

Fasting's neurobiological effects highlight its potential as a comprehensive strategy for enhancing brain health.

Cancer Shielding Secrets

Intermittent fasting's possible cancer-prevention benefits take the form of a multifaceted plan that combines several components to provide a strong defense against cancer (Nencioni et al., 2018):

- Through its protective effect on insulin sensitivity, intermittent fasting creates an environment that is less conducive to the development of cancer. One of the most important ways to stop the growth of cancer cells is to control the levels of insulin.

- Fasting protects against cancer by reducing chronic inflammation, which is known to play a role in the development of cancer. This alteration of the pro-cancerous milieu makes the growth of malignant cells less favorable.

- When it comes to protecting against cancer through intermittent fasting, the proverb "prevention is better than cure" holds true. The practice actively works to prevent the accumulation of damaged cells, which is a prelude to the development of cancer, by incorporating cellular repair processes.

- The cellular self-destruct mechanism known as apoptosis may be triggered by intermittent fasting. By guaranteeing damaged cells do not have the opportunity to develop into malignant entities, this procedure stops tumors from growing.

- Intermittent fasting appears to be a promising complementary strategy for lowering the risk of some cancers while further research explores its nuances.

It presents itself as a proactive strategy for cancer prevention due to its multifaceted effects on apoptosis, inflammation, cellular repair, and insulin sensitivity.

Age-Defying Cure

Starting an intermittent fasting journey reveals an age-defying potion that works at the molecular and cellular levels to address the core causes of aging:

- Imagine intermittent fasting as a watchful nanny that triggers autophagy to remove damaged cellular constituents. This cleansing process is similar to pressing a reset button because it lowers oxidative stress and creates an environment inside the cell that promotes cellular longevity.

- The reduction of oxidative stress, a silent force that adds to cellular wear and tear, is another aspect of the age-defying magic. Intermittent fasting acts as a protector, keeping cells resilient and alive by reducing oxidative stress.

- Our genes are woven under the influence of intermittent fasting. This genetic modification is a deep tactic that fosters resistance against age-related illnesses rather than merely a surface-level change. The genes turn into a road map for a longer, healthier life.

- The all-encompassing strategy of intermittent fasting to thwart the aging process is what makes it unique. Instead of being a quick cosmetic fix, it is a calculated plan that triggers a cascade of molecular and cellular changes. The rejuvenating power of intermittent fasting is not limited to superficial benefits; it goes deep.

When you adopt intermittent fasting, you are doing more than just changing your diet—you are participating in a life-changing, time-traveling practice. The age-defying elixir turns into an enduring friend that leads you to a life full of energy, resiliency, and an enduring cellular dance.

Metabolic Marvel

Starting this journey reveals a metabolic marvel—a dance of harmony between important hormones that alters the metabolic landscape of your body.

- The start of intermittent fasting is accompanied by a slow decline in insulin levels. This intentional decrease provides the body with the opportunity to switch from using glucose to burning fat stores for energy, which is an essential phase in metabolic transformation.

- Growth hormone assumes a prominent role, while insulin regresses gently. Increased growth hormone levels take on the role of the metabolic symphony's conductor, arranging a composition that burns fat while preserving muscle. A toned body and improved metabolic performance are the end results.

- Like a professional dancer, intermittent fasting increases insulin sensitivity in the body. This increased sensitivity makes sure that nutrients are used effectively, which promotes better metabolic health and fosters an environment in which the body flourishes.

- Insulin levels gradually drop, and the body starts to use fat reserves as a long-term source of energy. This deliberate use of fat reserves reshapes the body's contours and becomes a smart and successful weight management strategy.

- Beyond being a band-aid solution, intermittent fasting becomes a transformative and long-term strategy for changing the metabolic landscape of the body. Its metabolic dance facilitates better energy and overall metabolic health, in addition to helping with weight management.

The body experiences a metamorphic rhythm in the symphony of metabolic marvels orchestrated by intermittent fasting—a rhythm that redefines the fundamental essence of metabolic vitality, transcending aesthetics.

*****

So far on our journey, we have explored the complex terrain of intermittent fasting, revealing the wide range of fasting practices and their significant effects on health. The main lesson asks us to see intermittent fasting as a deliberate decision to change the way we relate to food and time rather than as a passing fad.

We took a close look at the various fasting techniques, such as the strict 16/8 plan, the provocative 5:2 diet, the reflective eat-stop-eat, and the unorthodox alternate-day fasting schedule. Every technique has its own rhythm, encouraging us to discover the one that fits best with our own way of life.

Now, we get ready to start a practical investigation by dipping our toes into the world of intermittent fasting as we turn the page to Chapter 2. Although there may be obstacles along the way, with the right information and tactics, we can conquer them and discover the keys to a more purposeful, harmonious, and healthy relationship with food, time, and well-being. Let's carry on with the fasting journey.

Chapter 2:

Getting Started With Intermittent

Fasting

Starting an intermittent fast is like embarking on a journey to become a more vibrant, healthier version of yourself. This is a commitment rather than merely a choice, an investment in your well-being that could have life-changing effects. As we explore this chapter, consider the journey ahead as a guide to successful intermittent fasting as well as pleasurable and long-lasting changes in lifestyle. Together, we will carefully navigate through the necessary steps to make sure that your journey starts with intention and purpose and prepares you for a refreshed you.

Assessing Personal Goals

The first and most important step in the world of intermittent fasting is to know your "why." What motivates you to embark on this journey? What goals for wellness and health drive your commitment? In order to discover your objectives and establish the foundation for a purposeful experience with intermittent fasting, let us start by addressing these questions through a self-exploration journey.

Understanding Your Why

Let's go through a few steps to help you find the answers you need to get started.

Establish Your Wellness and Health Objectives

Take a moment to clarify your main health goals before stepping foot in the world of intermittent fasting. Do you want to lose weight in order to get a more manageable body mass index? Is achieving stable blood sugar levels and better insulin sensitivity the main goal of metabolic health? Maybe you are considering cognitive enhancement as a way to improve your focus and mental clarity.

What is the reason for your fast?

Make Your Goals Specific

The power of clarity lies in specificity. Rather than aiming for a general objective such as "weight loss," specify the precise weight range you want to hit. Determine which markers to raise if the improvement is in metabolism. You could make a list of the cognitive abilities you hope to strengthen in order to meet your goals. With clarity, you can turn vague aspirations into specific goals and receive precise guidance for your intermittent fasting journey.

Acknowledge the Emotional Elements

Beyond achieving tangible goals, be aware of the emotional aspects of your journey. Are you looking for a renewed connection with your body, a sense of accomplishment, or an increase in confidence? Comprehending the affective undertones enhances your experience, turning it into a comprehensive undertaking that integrates mental and physical health.

Match Objectives to Lifestyle

Think about how your lifestyle fits with your goals for wellness and health. As there is no one-size-fits-all method for intermittent fasting, it is more sustainable to customize it to fit into your daily schedule. If you're a morning person, you might prefer a fasting window that aligns with your natural rhythm. You can incorporate intermittent fasting into your daily life with ease if you are aware of the dynamics of your lifestyle.

Consider the Long-Term Effects

And finally, consider how your goals will affect you later on. In what ways will reaching these goals improve your life in general? As a long-term lifestyle change, intermittent fasting offers numerous advantages over other temporary tactics. Imagine the long-term benefits of staying in line with your objectives. This will encourage you to stick with the intermittent fasting journey as a long-term investment in your health.

Remember that knowing your "why" will serve as your compass as you set out on this introspective journey, and use intermittent fasting as a guide. You can walk forward with purpose, and every step helps you achieve your goals of health and well-being when you have a clear destination in mind.

Setting Realistic Expectations

To create a lasting and fulfilling experience on this trip, you must consider it a marathon rather than a sprint. Let us explore the significance of establishing reasonable and attainable objectives, keeping in mind that intermittent fasting is a gradual process with significant long-term effects.

Adopt a Progressive Approach

Fasting intermittently promotes a gradual transformation as opposed to a quick cure. It is like planting a garden: With patience and care, the seeds you sow today will grow into something beautiful. Accept that change happens gradually and give your body time to adjust to the irregular fasting schedule without worrying about outcomes right away.

Acknowledge Little Victories

Appreciate the little triumphs you achieve along the way. These little victories, like following your preferred fasting regimen for a predetermined number of days or observing minor adjustments in your energy levels, are the foundation for bigger ones. Acknowledging and cherishing these little victories keeps you motivated and highlights the benefits of your experience with intermittent fasting.

Set Milestones and Adjust as Needed

Set attainable benchmarks that correspond with your overall objectives. These benchmarks act as checkpoints, enabling you to evaluate your progress and make the required corrections. If your first window of fasting proves to be challenging, consider gradually extending it as your body becomes acclimated to it. Being adaptable and resilient while navigating the terrain of intermittent fasting is ensured by having a flexible approach.

Acknowledge Individual Variability

Every person has a different journey. A number of variables, including lifestyle, health, and metabolism, affect how results vary. Pay attention to your personal journey and the positive changes you experience instead of comparing your progress to others'. A more positive outlook and a sense of self-compassion are fostered by embracing your uniqueness.

Put Your General Well-Being First

Shift your focus from purely outcome-based goals to prioritizing overall well-being. Intermittent fasting is not just about the numbers on a scale; it's a holistic approach to health. Observe an improvement in your mood, energy level, and mental clarity. These all-encompassing advantages enhance the positive experience and reaffirm the long-lasting effects of intermittent fasting on your health.

Stay Calm and Relentless

The key to a successful intermittent fasting journey is patience. Recognize that it will take some time for the body to adapt to the new eating habits. Long-term success is based on your ability to stick to your chosen fasting regimen in the face of obstacles. Have faith in the procedure, and keep in mind that each step you take now is a step toward long-term wellbeing.

As you prepare yourself for your journey of intermittent fasting, remember that mindful adjustments and steady progress are what pave the way to a healthier, more vibrant you. Setting realistic objectives and accepting that intermittent fasting is a gradual process will help you have a successful and long-lasting experience.

Choosing the Right Fasting Method

Navigating the diverse landscape of intermittent fasting methods is akin to choosing a personalized route map for your well-being. In this section, we will examine the alternative solutions discussed in Chapter 1. The goal? To help you determine which intermittent fasting plan best suits your preferences, lifestyle, and intended level of health.

What's Right For You?

The 16/8 Method

The 16/8 approach, sometimes referred to as time-restricted eating, calls for a 16-hour fasting window every day, followed by an 8-hour eating window. Those who like routine and structure in their daily lives tend to find this method appealing. When thinking about the 16/8 method, concentrate on how well it fits in with your health objectives (better metabolism and weight control). Consider how feasible an 8-hour eating window is for your everyday schedule. Determine how much longer you can fast while keeping in mind how it will affect your energy levels. Try a trial period where you track adherence and weight. Because the 16/8 method is both structured and flexible, it can be tailored to suit the preferences of each individual. The key to success is incorporating intermittent fasting into your daily routine in a way that is both beneficial and long-lasting.

The 5:2 Diet

The 5:2 diet involves introducing intermittent fasting by dividing a meal plan into two non-consecutive days of reduced calorie intake and five days of regular eating. You can discover the flexibility this approach provides and enjoy the advantages of fasting without having to commit to a daily fast. Determine whether the 5:2 approach works for you by evaluating your capacity to follow non-consecutive fasting days and your ability to control your calorie intake during fasting days. Think about your eating habits and whether the flexibility of this approach fits in with your dietary preferences. Try it out for a trial period to see how well it works and fits into your daily routine.

The Eat-Stop-Eat Fast

Eat-stop-eat calls for one or two 24-hour fasts per week. This technique offers an organized, sporadic approach to intermittent fasting. In evaluating whether this diet is for you, assess the feasibility of incorporating occasional, longer fasts into your daily routine. Consider whether the flexibility offered by the eat-stop-eat approach suits your lifestyle and delve into personal well-being, reflecting on how your body and mind respond to the intermittent rhythm of eat-stop-eat.

Alternate Day Fasting

The concept of ADF involves alternating between days when you eat normally and days when you consume very few calories or do not eat at all. Examine how well it fits with your health objectives when you give it some thought, paying particular attention to weight control and metabolic enhancements. Evaluate whether it makes sense for you to alternate fasting and regular days in your daily schedule and make sure they work well together. Determine how much you can tolerate fasting days and how they affect your overall health and energy levels. A trial period can provide information about adaptation, enabling changes to customize the strategy to your particular requirements. The ability of ADF to support a positive and long-lasting health journey depends on how well it fits your lifestyle, personal preferences, and health goals.

Taking Preferences and Lifestyle Into Account

Examine these techniques and see how each one fits into your daily schedule, professional obligations, and personal tastes. Your life should be improved, not worsened, by intermittent fasting. So, determine which approach best suits your lifestyle so that it becomes a fun and sustainable habit.

Remember, choosing the right intermittent fasting method entails more than just sticking to your health goals; it also means integrating yourself into your daily routine. The importance of lifestyle factors in selecting an intermittent fasting plan that will improve long-term outcomes will be covered once you go over your health objectives and a few other things to think about.

Daily Routine Dynamics

Think about the cadence of your everyday activities. If you eat breakfast first thing in the morning and are an early riser, the 16/8 method, with its early eating window, may work better for your natural flow. On the other hand, a later eating window could provide solace for night owls. Make sure your decision aligns with the rhythm of your day.

Syncing of Work Schedules

Consider how different intermittent fasting techniques fit into your work schedule. Fixed-hours workers may prefer 16/8 methods, while flexible schedules may find flexibility in the 5:2 diet or eat-stop-eat. You can make intermittent fasting a seamless part of your workday routine by making sure it works with your work commitments.

Harmony in Social Commitments

Our social lives are centered around meals and get-togethers most of the time. Consider how your chosen intermittent fasting strategy aligns with your societal responsibilities. While the 16/8 method's structure may offer consistency during social occasions, the flexibility of the 5:2 diet may allow for occasional indulgences. For long-term adherence, finding a balance that respects your social connections is essential.

Flexibility in Relation to Travel and Special Events

Intermittent fasting is dynamic, just like life itself. So, select a strategy that can adjust to life's unforeseen events, like trips or special occasions. Because intermittent fasting is flexible, it will enhance your lifestyle rather than place inflexible restrictions on it. Investigate techniques that allow you to modify fasting windows in accordance with particular situations.

Stress-Free Assimilation

A stress-free addition to your life should be intermittent fasting. Choose an approach that will work with your system as little as possible without interfering with your general health. Stress plays a big role in health, so pick a fasting strategy that fits in with your daily schedule to create a relaxed and harmonious atmosphere.

Respecting Circadian Rhythms

Think about timing your fasting windows to correspond with your body's circadian cycles. Eating in accordance with circadian rhythms may improve metabolic health, according to research. Investigate techniques that align with your body's internal clock in order to possibly increase the efficacy of your intermittent fasting regimen.

Trial and Adjustment Time Frame

Understand that it may take some trial and error to find the ideal fit. Try out various approaches and see how each fits into your way of life. This flexible strategy makes sure that intermittent fasting turns into a customized habit, increasing the chances of sustained success.

When you choose your intermittent fasting technique, consider it a cooperative effort between your daily life and your well-being objectives as you navigate lifestyle factors. Intermittent fasting becomes an essential and sustainable aspect of your lifestyle when it aligns with your routine, work schedule, and social obligations.

Handling Concerns With Periodic Fasting

Starting the journey of intermittent fasting may cause hesitation or concerns, and that is perfectly acceptable. Now, let's address common concerns, especially with ADF, with ideas and considerations to ease any fears you may have.

- First, let us examine the fundamentals of fasting on alternate days. With ADF, there are alternate days when you eat normally and days when you either consume very few calories or fast completely. This technique gives intermittent fasting a unique rhythm that promotes cellular and metabolic responses that enhance general health.

- Doubts regarding the severity of ADF are not unusual. Potential hunger pangs on fasting days and worries about maintaining such a pattern over time are just a few possible. It is necessary to first acknowledge these reservations in order to embark on an informed and purposeful intermittent fasting experience. Acknowledging these reservations is the first step toward an informed and mindful experience with intermittent fasting.

- Controlling hunger during days of fasting is one of the main issues. It is important to realize that feeling hungry is a common response to changing eating habits. However, by using strategies like drinking lots of water, enjoying herbal teas, and including nutrient-dense foods on non-fasting days, a more manageable transition can be accomplished.

- Making sure there are enough nutrients, particularly on days when you are consuming fewer calories, is another concern. In order to make up for any possible nutrient gaps, ADF stresses the significance of eating foods high in nutrients on non-fasting days. Maintaining general health requires balancing the nutritional value of your meals during the times you eat them.

- The time needed to adjust to intermittent fasting should be taken into account. Your body can adjust to the new pattern and minimize difficulties by gradually extending fasting periods and starting with less restrictive fasting windows.

- With ADF and other intermittent fasting, you will exhibit individual differences in response when compared with another. What fits one person perfectly might need to be adjusted for another. Recognize and value your individual journey, and remember that intermittent fasting techniques can be customized to meet your requirements and comfort level.

- It is wise to seek professional advice if worries continue or worsen. Speaking with a registered dietitian or other healthcare professional can address specific health concerns and offer individualized insights. Your health comes first, and expert guidance guarantees a successful and safe intermittent fasting experience.

- If your concerns about ADF are too great, you might want to look into some of the other intermittent fasting strategies we covered earlier, like the 16/8 method or the 5:2 diet. Long-term success requires finding a method that fits more harmoniously with your comfort zone and lifestyle.

You give yourself the power to decide whether or not a certain method of fasting is a good fit for your intermittent fasting journey by admitting and resolving any concerns you may have. Keep in mind that your health comes first and that you can customize an intermittent fasting plan to suit your needs and tastes, thanks to its flexibility.

Advice for a Smooth Transition

It is an exciting first step toward better health to begin an intermittent fast, and understanding the significance of staying hydrated will help you navigate the shift with ease. It's time to look at the crucial relationship between hydration and the length of a fast, as well as practical tips on how to maintain optimal fluid balance and use hydration to your advantage when attempting intermittent fasting.

How Important Is Hydration?

Adequate hydration is the cornerstone of good health, and fasting periods highlight how crucial this is. Water is necessary for many physiological functions, such as digestion and body temperature regulation. In order to navigate intermittent fasting successfully, one must comprehend the importance of staying hydrated.

- It is important to drink as much water as possible when eating or not fasting. This is to make up for any fluids lost while fasting. Although eight glasses of water a day is a general recommendation, individual requirements may differ depending on factors such as activity level and climate.

- Incorporate herbal teas and infusions into your hydration routine to make it better. In addition to encouraging you to drink more water, they can provide a variety of flavors to improve your fasting experience. Choosing herbal teas, such as chamomile or peppermint, is a great idea. Decaffeinated teas ensure that you stay hydrated without becoming energized.

- Electrolyte balance must be maintained, especially during extended fasts. Consider including foods or supplements high in electrolytes to improve hydration. Nuts, seeds, and leafy greens are natural sources of electrolytes. However, you should consult a healthcare professional before starting any supplement regimen.

- Avoiding overhydration is just as important as staying hydrated. Excessive water consumption can cause electrolyte levels to drop, which can result in hyponatremia. Pay attention to your body's signals and drink water in moderation throughout the day to avoid consuming too much at once.

- Look into drinks that are suitable for intermittent fasting that will keep you hydrated without causing you to break your fast. Black coffee, plain water, and unsweetened herbal teas are all great options. Try drinks that fit your fasting objectives and personal tastes.

- In order to practice mindful water intake, you should consistently sip water throughout the day as opposed to consuming large amounts at once. This method guarantees a continuous flow of fluids, promoting general health and reducing the possibility of discomfort during fasting periods.

- Above all, pay attention to your body's signals. Being aware of this cue will help you stay well-hydrated because thirst is a natural indicator of dehydration. In case you notice any signs of dehydration, like lightheadedness or dark urine, make sure you rehydrate as soon as possible.

When you align your intermittent fasting journey with hydration, water becomes more than just a drink; it becomes an ally. Allow water to play a crucial role in supporting your fasting experience and facilitating a smooth transition to a more vibrant and healthier version of yourself.

Nutrient-Rich Foods: Nourishing Your Body During Eating Windows

The intricate motions of intermittent fasting highlight the significance of eating windows that are rich in nutrients. These foods not only sate your hunger but also supply your body with essential vitamins and minerals, which are the building blocks of overall health. Let us look at the importance of eating meals high in nutrients and explore dietary choices that enhance both your overall health and your degree of satisfaction.

The Fundamentals of Nutrient Density

Foods high in nutrients provide a potent dose of essential nutrients relative to their calorie content. By including these foods in your diet, you can be certain that each meal meets your body's cellular needs for nourishment as well as your energy requirements.

- Make meals that balance the three macronutrients—carbs, fats, and proteins—a priority. This equilibrium helps control blood sugar levels, maintains muscle health, and gives long-lasting energy. For a well-balanced and filling plate, think about adding lean proteins, healthy fats, and complex carbohydrates.

- A wealth of vitamins, minerals, and antioxidants can be found in vegetables, making them nutritional powerhouses. To guarantee a wide range of nutrients, embrace a colorful variety. Various vegetables such as leafy greens, colorful bell peppers, cruciferous vegetables, and root vegetables offer distinct advantages. A plate should be visually appealing and varied.

- In addition to sating hunger, lean proteins aid in the upkeep and repair of muscles. Tofu and legumes are very good options. Including foods high in protein at mealtimes improves satiety and helps you avoid consuming too many calories during eating windows.

- Add good fats to your diet to help maintain overall health and provide long-lasting energy. Excellent providers of monounsaturated and polyunsaturated fats are avocados, nuts, seeds, and olive oil. In addition to giving a feeling of fullness, these fats aid in the absorption of nutrients.

- If you want a longer-lasting energy release, go for whole grains rather than refined ones. Whole grains are high in vitamins, minerals, and fiber. Examples of these include brown rice, quinoa, and oats. They help keep blood sugar levels stable and support good digestive health.

Conscientious Portion Management

Although foods high in nutrients are good for you, eating in moderation guarantees a balanced diet. Savor every bite and pay attention to your body's signals of hunger and fullness. Portion sizes that are balanced discourage overindulgence and foster a healthy connection with food.

Include beverages in the concept of nutrient density. Choose nutrient-dense drinks like infused water, green tea, and herbal teas. These options offer extra vitamins and antioxidants in addition to helping you stay hydrated. Also, make sure your nutrient-dense meals fit your dietary requirements and preferences. There is a wide range of nutrient-rich options to meet your needs, regardless of whether you follow a plant-based diet, follow particular nutritional guidelines, or have dietary restrictions.

By consuming a wide variety of nutrient-dense foods, you can turn your mealtimes into occasions for health and nourishment. Accept the wide range of healthy options available to you, and turn every meal into an occasion to celebrate your overall health and well-being as well as your journey toward intermittent fasting.

Organizing Meals

Meal planning within your allocated eating windows is the most vibrant way to paint the picture of your intermittent fasting journey. Creating meals that suit your dietary preferences and goals becomes a thoughtful and artistic process. Let's get into the nuances of meal planning with the benefits as well as four tips that will help you transform your food choices into well-balanced, satisfying masterpieces.

The Benefits of Meal Planning

- Meal planning is a deliberate process that helps you arrange and structure your meals so they meet your nutritional goals. This procedure entails carefully weighing the components, serving sizes, and general meal composition for every meal within the parameters of your allotted eating windows.

- Meal planning success depends on achieving a strategic balance of macronutrients, or proteins, fats, and carbohydrates. So, always ensure that these essential ingredients are included in a balanced combination in your meals. This balance not only encourages satiety but also optimal energy levels and encourages overall well-being.

- A range of fruits, vegetables, whole grains, and lean proteins should be included. Why? Well, this vivid palette guarantees a wide range of vital vitamins and minerals and improves the sensory experience of eating.

- Making thoughtful food choices is an essential part of meal planning. It entails understanding portion sizes so that you can have a filling, well-balanced meal without going overboard. To determine the proper portion sizes for proteins, carbs, and fats, use visual cues like plate division.

- Planning meals also entails batch cooking and preparation. So, you will need to set aside particular times to organize and prepare meals ahead of time. You can make some dishes in larger quantities with batch cooking, which is convenient and guarantees that you have nutrient-dense options available when you want them.

Tips for Personalization According to Your Preferences

- Make sure that the meal planning techniques you use suit your dietary requirements and preferences.

- Adapt your meal plans to suit your specific nutritional requirements and increase overall enjoyment, regardless of whether you have food sensitivities, adhere to dietary guidelines, or follow a particular eating philosophy.

- Think about including snacks that are high in nutrients. These can help you eat more mindfully by providing you with a nutritional and energy boost in between meals. Choose things like sliced veggies with hummus or Greek yogurt with berries and nuts.

- Arrange your meals so that your fluid intake is strategically coordinated. Drink water slowly in between bites to achieve a harmonious harmony.

Consider meal planning as an artistic and liberating endeavor as you embark on your intermittent fasting journey. These techniques are meant to help you achieve your nutritional objectives as well as transform your meals into satisfying and nourishing experiences. Gaining proficiency in meal planning allows you to turn every mealtime into a chance to enjoy well-balanced, gratifying, and nutritious food.

*****

The information above serves as your reliable compass as you approach intermittent fasting, providing direction through the crucial phases of preparation, method choice, and the smooth transition of fasting into your regular routine. Your chosen course is an intentional journey toward transformation rather than just a commitment.

Always look beyond; think of intermittent fasting as a journey that will involve purpose, decision-making, and personal development as you embark on it. Watch as a new chapter opens up for you, one in which every window of opportunity for growth during your fasting period becomes an opportunity to grow and improve yourself. Now, as you navigate the complex terrain of intermittent fasting with purpose and intention, get ready to be the architect of your own transformation. One fasting window at a time, the path ahead promises not only health gains but also a profound metamorphosis.

Chapter 3:

Overcoming Common Challenges

Starting an intermittent fasting journey can be a life-changing experience, but all life-changing experiences come with difficulties. This chapter lays out the map of the road ahead and covers common obstacles you may encounter on your journey to successful intermittent fasting. You will be armed with strategies to overcome obstacles, just as an experienced traveler prepares for the ups and downs of the journey. Every obstacle becomes a chance for development, from controlling hunger and navigating social situations to overcoming energy slumps and adjusting to different body types. Come, let's move forward with the subtle art of conquering everyday obstacles so that your intermittent fasting practice stays steady, intentional, and ultimately successful. Let us go on this journey.

Dealing With Hunger

Understanding Fasting-Induced Hunger

One of the common threads in the complex pattern of intermittent fasting is hunger. But not all hunger is equal, and to successfully navigate this part of the journey, you must grasp the subtleties of hunger brought on by fasting. Let's set out to discern between the physiological hunger that comes with fasting times and the psychological or habitual hunger that could skew our understanding.

What Causes Hunger During a Fast?

Hunger that develops during a fast is a natural reaction to not eating during certain times. In contrast to emotional or habitual hunger, which can be brought on by outside stimuli or emotional states, hunger brought on by fasting is a natural byproduct of the body's adjustment to a new eating schedule. The hunger that is brought on by fasting is frequently a slow, subtle sensation that indicates that your body is ready for food but without the urgency of emotional or impulsive eating. Ghrelin, known as the "hunger hormone," is a key player in informing the brain when you're hungry. The hormonal shifts that take place during fasting, such as variations in ghrelin levels, affect how hungry you feel. However, note that your body adapts and that, as it gets used to the new eating pattern, hunger that is brought on by fasting tends to decrease. In order to give your body the opportunity to adapt to and develop a healthy relationship with hunger cues, persistence and patience are essential.

It is possible to overcome hunger issues as you approach nourishment while eating with mindfulness and intention. When navigating the ups and downs of hunger during an intermittent fast, see it as an opportunity to strengthen your relationship with your body's natural wisdom rather than a challenge. This realization is the first step in learning how to manage your hunger, and it lays a strong foundation for an enjoyable and meaningful experience with intermittent fasting.

Always try to make a clear distinction between cravings that originate from emotional triggers, external stimuli, or conditioned responses and true hunger. You can respond to true hunger with nourishing choices and mindfully address cravings when you are mindful of your body's signals.

Strategies for Managing Hunger: Navigating the Fasting Windows With Ease

As you progress through your intermittent fasting journey, controlling your hunger during fasting windows becomes a skill. Once you have mastered it, you can turn potential discomfort into a powerful and seamless experience. Let's go over doable strategies for managing and lessening hunger pangs so that your journey is emotionally and cognitively stimulating in addition to being physically fulfilling.

- Make staying hydrated your top priority as a basic method to control your hunger when fasting. Water consumption enhances general well-being in addition to promoting a full feeling. Drink water frequently throughout the day to maintain proper hydration.

- Calorie-free herbal teas can provide solace during periods of fasting. Try experimenting with different herbal teas, like ginger, chamomile, or peppermint; these will help you stay hydrated and may also help you feel less hungry.

- To combat hunger in between meals, think about including nutrient-dense snacks in your eating window at strategic intervals. You can be satiated without sacrificing your fasting objectives with foods like sliced veggies with hummus, Greek yogurt with berries, or a handful of nuts.

- When breaking your fast, practice mindful eating and place a strong emphasis on savoring every bite. Eating mindfully helps you develop a stronger bond with your food, which increases satisfaction and lowers the risk of overindulging because of lingering hunger.

- Increase the length of the fasting period gradually so that your body can get used to it. As your body adjusts to the rhythm of intermittent fasting, start with a comfortable fasting window and gradually extend it over time through experimentation.

- Prepare meals that emphasize fullness by incorporating a harmony of macronutrients, such as complex carbohydrates, healthy fats, and proteins. In addition to giving long-lasting energy, a well-balanced meal helps induce fullness, which reduces hunger in between fasting periods.

- During fasting periods, use exercise or light physical activity as a diversion from hunger. Engaging in physical activity, such as yoga, stretching, or brisk walking, can help you focus on things other than food and improve your general health.

- To control stress-induced hunger, try progressive muscle relaxation or deep breathing exercises. Stress can exacerbate feelings of hunger, and integrating calming practices can positively impact both mental well-being and hunger perception.

- Lastly, maintain a journal to monitor your hunger patterns and pinpoint possible triggers. Use this information to modify your meal plans, water intake tactics, or fasting schedule in accordance with your own responses and requirements.

You give yourself the ability to proactively control your hunger and transform possible obstacles into chances for personal development by adding these tactics to your toolkit for intermittent fasting. Keep in mind that controlling your hunger is a personal journey, and you can customize these strategies to fit your own tastes and experiences. Accept that your relationship with hunger is changing as you easily navigate the fasting windows; this is evidence of your resiliency and dedication to having a positive intermittent fasting experience.

The Role of Hydration, Herbal Teas, and Nutrient-Dense Foods in Curbing Hunger and Promoting Satiety

Hydration, herbal teas, and nutrient-dense foods play a crucial role in controlling hunger and promoting satiety during intermittent fasting. These elements provide both physical and psychological support, making them more than just companions on your journey but formidable allies. Let us explore the distinct roles that each plays in reducing hunger and making sure that your fasting periods are not only observed but also looked forward to with a feeling of satisfaction.

- Water becomes your most important weapon against hunger when you are fasting. In addition to contributing to a feeling of fullness, hydration is essential for many biological processes. Drink enough water throughout the day to prevent dehydration and promote general well-being, especially during fasting periods.

- Herbal teas provide a soothing and hydrating substitute during fasting because they are low in calories and frequently high in antioxidants. While chamomile tea has a mild calming effect, peppermint tea can ease digestive discomfort with its calming qualities. Try a variety of herbal teas to determine which ones are your favorites for being both hydrating and satiating.

- With their abundance of vitamins, minerals, and satiating qualities, nutrient-dense foods are the unsung heroes in your battle against hunger. Include foods like leafy greens, nuts, seeds, lean proteins, complex carbohydrates, whole grains, fiber, and good fats in your daily meals.

Strategic Meal Timing and Composition

To maximize satiety, space out your nutrient-dense meals throughout your eating window. A consistent feeling of fullness is facilitated by balancing the macronutrients (carbs, fats, and proteins) in each meal, which also helps to avoid sudden spikes and crashes in blood sugar levels.

Hydration Without Water

Try other hydrating drinks besides water, like citrus fruit slices or water infused with fresh herbs. A dash of natural flavors adds another level of sensory satisfaction to hydration while also making it look more appealing.

Make drinking herbal tea a ritual part of your mindful eating routine. Take in the flavor and scent of the tea with your senses, fostering a mindful experience that will enhance your overall enjoyment of the fasting process.

Give pre-fasting hydration first priority to ensure ideal fluid balance during fasting periods. After a fast, hydrate yourself with hydrating drinks and eat foods high in nutrients to help your body recover by replenishing electrolytes.

You can proactively address hunger during fasting by being aware of the many benefits of drinking plenty of water, drinking herbal teas, and eating foods high in nutrients. As you incorporate these components into your intermittent fasting regimen, keep in mind that the goal is not only to endure hunger but also to embrace it, knowing that your allies are helping you become a more resilient, nourished, and satisfied version of yourself.

Mindful Eating Practices

The practice of mindful eating shines as a beacon of balance in the fast-paced rhythm of modern life. It becomes a profound journey of connection with your body's innate wisdom and goes beyond simple eating. Using mindful eating practices makes every meal a meaningful and mindful experience as you navigate the waters of intermittent fasting. Let's see how you can develop this mindful approach and strengthen your relationship with your body's signals of hunger and fullness.

- Start every meal by taking a moment to be still and focus on the here and now. Remove all sources of distraction, including electronics, and establish a special area for eating.

- Take in the flavors, textures, and colors of your food to stimulate your senses. Eat more slowly and deliberately, enjoying every bite with conscious thought.

- In addition to making eating more enjoyable, focusing on the flavors and textures of your food helps your body recognize when it has been fed.

- Throughout the meal, pay attention to your body's cues about hunger and fullness.

- Mindful chewing involves savoring the taste and texture of each bite, allowing the digestive process to begin in the mouth.

- Close your eyes briefly to heighten taste sensations or bring awareness to the sounds associated with your meal. This sensory immersion elevates the act of eating from a routine to a mindful exploration.

- Develop an attitude of thankfulness by appreciating the path that each component took to get to your plate. Eating becomes a more holistic experience that goes beyond the physical with this practice.

- Recognize the difference between emotional and physical cravings so that you can make decisions that are in line with your well-being in response to each.

- Create a calm and welcoming dining space to set the tone for mindful eating.

- Select a serene location, set beautiful table settings, and surround yourself with things that make the experience better all around.

- Include mindful eating practices in your daily routine, such as giving yourself a moment of appreciation before meals or taking a quick moment to reflect afterward.

- Regular mindful eating cultivates a healthy relationship with food, transforming eating from a practical activity into a holy ritual of sustenance.

By incorporating these mindful eating practices into your intermittent fasting journey, you can develop a positive relationship with food in addition to providing your body with nourishment. Every meal turns into an intentional celebration of nourishment, allowing you to establish a closer relationship with your body's complex signals of hunger, fullness, and satisfaction. Let eating become a transformative experience that enhances your physical and spiritual well-being as you begin this mindful exploration.

Modifications to Lifestyle

Handling Social Situations With Comfort

Starting an intermittent fasting journey is more than just making a personal commitment; it also involves navigating the social environments that influence how we interact with each other on a daily basis. As you adopt this life-changing approach, good communication becomes essential to securing sympathy and encouragement from loved ones, coworkers, and friends. Let's see how you can confidently explain your fasting regimen and turn any possible social obstacles into chances for communication and understanding.

- Learn about the benefits of intermittent fasting first. This will enable you to confidently and clearly communicate your decisions.

- Give accurate information about intermittent fasting while highlighting its benefits for overall health and wellness. A well-informed explanation can help debunk misconceptions and advance understanding.

- Choose a time and location that works for you to inform people about your fasting regimen.

- Select moments when you can talk openly in order to minimize outside distractions and encourage focused conversation.

- Share the private motivations behind your choice to follow an intermittent fasting schedule. Expressing your reasons enables others to understand the deeper meaning underlying your decision, whether it is for your health, well-being, or the accomplishment of particular objectives.

- Instead of being a strict or constrictive way of living, remember that intermittent fasting is a flexible strategy that can be adjusted to fit a variety of social contexts and occasions.

- Express to those who are close to you your need for their understanding and support. Indicate that you value their support in fostering an atmosphere that supports your health objectives and that your decision to practice intermittent fasting is a personal one.

- Seek opportunities to engage in social events that coincide with your fasting schedule.

- Make suggestions for different kinds of social gatherings that do not center around meals, like get-togethers outside, coffee dates, or occasions where fasting can be easily incorporated.

- Encourage an environment that is transparent so that family and friends can feel free to ask questions. To help others understand your point of view and perhaps spark their interest in intermittent fasting, foster curiosity, and have conversations.

- Explain how your sporadic fasting has or is improving your life and provides you with advantages. Setting a good example for others can inspire them, and if you do so consistently, they might eventually start to accept your lifestyle choices.

- You open the door to your social circle's understanding and support when you approach social and lifestyle adjustments with open communication and a positive outlook. Keep in mind that having an open conversation with others enables them to understand the significance of your intermittent fasting journey in relation to your overall well-being. Effective communication is a two-way street.

Approaches to Social Events

This is something we all dread when we begin a fast, but worry not because we can overcome every challenge.

Yes, our lives are interwoven with social events, and yet, it is possible to enjoy and smoothly follow your fasting schedule while attending them. Here are some useful tips to help you stick to your intermittent fasting regimen and handle social situations with grace:

- When possible, schedule your eating time to align with social gatherings. You can participate in the communal dining experience during the event as long as it does not conflict with your scheduled fasting hours.

- Arrange or propose social events that coincide with your fasting period. Fasting can be easily incorporated into other activities or events that do not center around meals.

- Tell the event organizer or attendees that you plan to fast intermittently. Giving advance notice enables people to be aware of your dietary restrictions and might even encourage thoughtful meal-planning decisions.

- When attending events, prioritize socializing over eating. Take part in activities, have meaningful conversations, and enjoy each other's company without putting too much emphasis on the food at the event.

- Make sure you stay hydrated when attending social gatherings without food. To stay hydrated and honor your fasting window, choose herbal teas, water, or other non-caloric beverages.

- Bring little, suitable-for-fasting snacks so you have them on hand for events. When it comes to discreetly maintaining energy levels without drawing attention to your fasting choices, nuts, seeds, and other portable options can be a great option.

- When choosing meals to eat during your fasting window, make sure they fit your dietary requirements.

- In order to adhere to the guidelines of your intermittent fasting plan, choose foods that are high in nutrients, such as vegetables and lean proteins.

- Eat mindfully if you choose to eat during a social gathering. Savor each bite, eat in small portions, and pay attention to your body's signals of fullness. You can take part and maintain your commitment at the same time by practicing mindful eating.

- Look into possibilities for non-eating-related activities. Instead of focusing on food, suggest activities like game nights, book club meetings, or outdoor excursions as ways to foster social connections.

- Accept change and do not hesitate to modify your fasting regimen for unique events. Periodic adaptability ensures that your journey of intermittent fasting is flexible enough to adjust to social dynamics without becoming too rigid or stressful.

- Do not feel guilty or judge yourself when you enjoy the social interaction to the fullest. Finding harmony between social gatherings and intermittent fasting is key, and appreciating the occasion for what it is helps to create a positive and long-lasting approach.

You can attend social gatherings with assurance if you put these tactics into practice because you will be able to handle them in a way that respects your commitment to intermittent fasting. Finding a balance that lets you maintain your commitment to your health and well-being objectives while still enjoying the richness of social interactions is crucial.

Incorporating Fasting Into Daily Life

Flexibility and thoughtful preparation are necessary to successfully incorporate intermittent fasting into different aspects of your daily life (Shields, 2020). Here are some suggestions for easily integrating intermittent fasting into your varied lifestyle, whether you are juggling work obligations, taking vacations, or enjoying leisure activities:

- Make sure that the times you fast correspond with the hours you work. If at all possible, schedule your fasting periods during off-peak hours to avoid interfering with your professional obligations.

- Arrange your workspace with options that are suitable for fasting. To support your fasting routine during work hours, keep nutrient-dense snacks, herbal teas, and non-caloric beverages on hand.

- Arrange your meals in a way that best fits your work schedule. Plan your meals for breaks or lunchtime to ensure that you can still eat healthfully and meet your fasting objectives.

- Maximize the duration of your fasting window by utilizing the travel time. Whether you are traveling for business or pleasure, see these times as chances to extend your fast and keep your routine.

- Carry lightweight, non-perishable snacks with you for any time you need to go. Having foods that are suitable for fasting on hand guarantees that you can follow your eating windows even when traveling or engaging in leisure activities.

- Choose foods and recipes that fit your preferences for intermittent fasting. Discover commonly available options that can be adjusted for fasting, making it simpler to stick to your routine while indulging in a variety of culinary experiences.

- Schedule your free time around the times you fast. Whether it is a day of leisure or a weekend getaway, schedule your fasting to work in harmony with your favorite activities.

- Track and organize your schedule with apps designed for intermittent fasting. Apps can help you stay consistent in many areas of your daily life by tracking fasting windows, sending you reminders, and providing insightful data.

- Inform the people you are traveling with about your decision to observe an intermittent fast. Clear communication promotes understanding and enables group planning that takes into account everyone's preferences.

- Make sure you stay hydrated when you are having fun. When hiking, touring, or enjoying leisure activities, make it a priority to stay hydrated by drinking water or other non-caloric beverages. This will promote your overall health.

- Be willing to modify your fasting plans on special occasions. Maintaining consistency is important, but occasionally being flexible during special occasions or festivities guarantees you can participate completely without feeling constrained.

- Consider sporadic fasting as a flexible and conscientious way of living. Because life is dynamic, you should embrace the fact that intermittent fasting should enrich rather than detract from your daily experiences.

You can adapt intermittent fasting to your daily routine with ease if you plan ahead and embrace flexibility. Whether at work, on vacation, or during leisure activities, the secret is to develop a personalized, sustainable strategy that improves your general well-being.

Striking a Balance Between Regularity and Adaptability

It takes consistency to continue your intermittent fasting journey, but you do not have to avoid social situations in order to do so. Flexibility and adaptability become the cornerstones that ensure your fasting goals encourage social interactions and prevent you from feeling isolated. These elements work well together as follows:

- Be flexible with your meal schedule when attending social events. If necessary, reschedule your fasting to coincide with shared meals so that you can attend important events without feeling excluded from society. Plan ahead and allow some flexibility in your intermittent fasting schedule.

- Allocate specific days or times for a more laid-back attitude so you can go to social gatherings without feeling constrained by a strict fasting regimen.

- Discuss your decision to observe an intermittent fast with your loved ones in an open and sincere manner. Since open communication fosters understanding, you are less likely to feel alone when others begin to support you on your health journey.

- Engage your loved ones in your journey by discussing intermittent fasting with them. Those closest to you are more likely to respect your decisions and create a shared experience rather than a lonely one when they are aware of the guiding principles and benefits.

- Choose a place for social gatherings where fasting options are available. By choosing restaurants with a wide range of menu options, including ones that fit within your fasting window, you can be sure that you can attend social events without breaking your fast.

- When sharing meals with others, eat with awareness. Adopting mindful eating techniques allows you to savor your food and interact with others during your eating window, creating a harmonious balance between regularity and flexibility.

- Embrace the occasional treat with gusto. Recognize that, with the occasional exception for special occasions, long-term intermittent fasting is necessary to maintain your overall health.

impacted by changes in fasting practices; patience is essential during this transition.

- Recognize how important staying hydrated is in preventing low energy. Getting enough fluids during fasting periods is crucial because dehydration can exacerbate feelings of fatigue.

- Ensure electrolyte equilibrium, particularly when fasting for extended periods of time. In order to maintain energy levels and avert potential imbalances, think about including foods or supplements high in electrolytes.

- Examine the timing of your nutrients during the eating window. Strategically distributing nutrients during the meal can help maintain energy levels and avoid abrupt drops.

- During the fast, pay attention to the cues your body gives you. Seeking professional advice is advisable to ensure overall well-being if persistent low energy levels are accompanied by other forms of discomfort.

- Be willing to adapt your fasting techniques as needed. Extended periods of low energy might be an indication that you should review and maybe adjust your fasting schedule to better fit your body's requirements.

- Consult a professional if necessary. Seeking advice from a nutritionist or healthcare provider can offer tailored insights and suggestions if energy lows continue or are concerning.

Understanding the dynamics of energy fluctuations will enable you to make informed decisions about intermittent fasting. Understanding the variables at work enables you to make wise adjustments so that your energy levels and the objectives of your journey toward intermittent fasting are in harmony.

Maintaining Optimal Vitality Along With Techniques for Overcoming Depression

During intermittent fasting, combating energy lows requires calculated methods that maximize nutrient intake. The following are practical methods to maintain high levels of energy during your fast:

- Place a focus on nutrient-dense foods when preparing meals. Include a range of fruits, vegetables, and whole grains to supply a range of vital nutrients that support long-term energy.

- Maintain balanced macronutrient ratios in your meals. Aim for a balance of healthy fats, proteins, and carbs to encourage a prolonged, steady release of energy.

- Plan your dietary intake of nutrients to coincide with the times you eat. Spread out nutrient-dense foods over several meals to avoid focusing all of your energy in one sitting and to avoid energy crashes.

- Mindfully include energy-boosting snacks.

- Snack on foods that combine carbohydrates and proteins, like yogurt or a piece of fruit with nuts, for a rapid and long-lasting energy boost.

- Make use of water to increase your energy. Drinking water, herbal teas, and other non-caloric beverages will help you maintain an ideal fluid balance, which can help prevent fatigue.

- When observing extended fasts, give careful thought to food options that are high in electrolytes. To maintain hydration and energy levels, include foods and drinks that contain electrolytes, such as coconut water or electrolyte supplements.

- Consume caffeine mindfully for a controlled energy boost. Restrict your caffeine intake to prevent overstimulation, and for a steady and gradual energy boost, go for sources like black coffee or green tea.

- Within your eating window, experiment with small, frequent meals. By breaking up your meals into smaller, more frequent servings, you can help keep your blood sugar levels stable and avoid energy crashes.

- Make whole grains a part of your diet. Complex carbohydrates found in whole grains help you feel fuller for longer periods of time when you fast.

- Adapt nutrient choices to align with personal preferences. Make your meals special by adding foods you love and making sure they support long-term energy and general health.

- Make dietary choices high in protein. Protein is an important part of meals and snacks because it helps curb hunger and offers a sustained energy source.

- Make sure a variety of nutrients are included in your meal plans. Including a variety of nutrients in your diet improves general health and vitality, which in turn boosts energy levels.

You can build a nutritional base that sustains energy levels during intermittent fasting by putting these strategies into practice. Adapt these strategies to your tastes and way of life to create a balanced experience that improves your physical and mental health during your fast.

Energy Optimization

To sustain energy levels during the intermittent fasting journey, a thoughtful approach to meal timing, hydration, and balanced macronutrient intake is needed. We looked at this briefly before, but now, let's take a deeper look at the importance of each element.

Proper Macronutrient Balance

- Essentially, the main source of energy is carbohydrates. To provide a consistent release of energy, choose complex carbohydrates found in whole grains, fruits, and vegetables.

- Proteins are necessary for both satiety and muscle repair. Incorporate protein sources that are low in fat, such as legumes and tofu, to sustain energy levels and promote general health.

- Fats provide enduring energy. Include heart-healthy fats from nuts, seeds, avocados, and olive oil to promote fullness and maintain energy levels.

Hydration as the Fundamental

- Maintaining proper hydration is essential for long-term energy. Water is essential for many body processes, including the metabolism of energy. Make sure you drink enough water at the appropriate times during the fasting and eating windows.

- Eat foods high in electrolytes, particularly during extended fasting or vigorous exercise. Potassium, sodium, and magnesium are examples of electrolytes that support energy balance and hydration.

Time Your Meals Wisely

- Recognize that there may be a natural decline in energy during fasting windows. Before starting a fast, choose meals that are high in nutrients to give you long-lasting energy.

- Arrange mealtimes in a thoughtful manner throughout the window. Aim for a macronutrient balance to prevent abrupt changes in energy levels. To avoid energy dips and maintain stable blood sugar levels, think about eating smaller, more frequent meals.

- Always remember that nutrition should come before and after exercise. Modify nutrient consumption based on when you exercise. Before working out, eating a well-balanced meal or snack that includes both protein and carbs can increase energy levels. Prioritize a high-protein, high-carb meal after your workout for recovery and long-lasting energy.

Combination of Elements

- Stable blood sugar levels are a result of balanced macronutrients, which help to minimize swings in energy.

- The body's circadian rhythm and metabolism are supported by carefully planning when to eat. Meal timing that coincides with times when energy demand is highest improves overall energy use.

- Maintaining adequate hydration promotes effective nutrient transport, which facilitates the body's use of macronutrients for long-term energy.

Customization and Flexibility

- Be aware that different people may react differently to different macronutrient ratios, hydration requirements, and meal timings. Adjust your strategy according to how your body reacts to various tactics.

- Modify your hydration and macronutrient distribution plans in accordance with the particular intermittent fasting technique you employ. Various techniques might call for subtle strategies to maximize energy levels.

Essentially, the foundation of sustained energy during the intermittent fasting journey is the combination of strategically timed meals, hydration, and balanced macronutrients. Through comprehension and customization of these components to your personal requirements, you develop a comprehensive strategy that promotes life, improves output, and upholds general health.

Embracing Diversity: Navigating Bio-Individuality in Intermittent Fasting

It is crucial to acknowledge and value your bio-individuality when on an intermittent fast. The concept of "bio-individuality" recognizes that everyone is different, possessing unique physiological and genetic traits that affect how we react to different lifestyle interventions, such as intermittent fasting. Now, let us explore how important it is to comprehend bio-individuality in relation to intermittent fasting.

Individualized Fasting Responses

Individual metabolic responses during fasting vary, which affects your energy levels, mental clarity, and hormone-induced adaptation periods. Nutrition is heavily influenced by bio-individuality, which allows you to customize your nutrient intake based on your dietary preferences and sensitivities. It takes awareness of various transition periods to help with the complex process of adjusting to intermittent fasting and prevent any physical strain. Considerations related to lifestyle, such as work schedules and sleep patterns, emphasize how important it is to integrate fasting practices with daily routines harmoniously. Since everyone's experience with fasting's impact on exercise performance varies, a personalized plan based on individual preferences is needed. Psychological elements—like stress management during fasting— emphasize how particular this health regimen is. Understanding bio-individuality is the first step in determining personalized durations that suit individual needs, so tailoring fasting windows is an essential component of this process. Genetic influences influence the body's response to intermittent fasting, guiding tailored approaches for optimal health outcomes (Wang & Wu, 2022).

Guiding Principles for Personalization

To guarantee a customized intermittent fasting experience, you must reflect on your own reactions, evaluate yourself on a regular basis to make necessary adjustments and consult medical professionals for specialized advice, especially if you have particular health issues. Accepting the strength in differences and building self-assurance in navigating intermittent fasting within the framework of personal uniqueness are essential to empowering through diversity. Acknowledging varied reactions in a nurturing environment fosters shared experiences and group development.

Essentially, the key to successfully navigating intermittent fasting is customizing the practice to your physiological and lifestyle characteristics, which fosters empowerment and overall well-being.

Empowering Self-Awareness With a Personalized Approach to Intermittent Fasting

Handling the ever-changing world of intermittent fasting calls for a customized strategy based on self-awareness. Starting a mindful eating journal and recording meals, fasting intervals, and any emotional or physical reactions is the first step in this journey. It becomes essential to be able to distinguish between genuine hunger and emotional cues, so you should experiment with different fasting windows and track changes in your hunger patterns.

Frequent energy evaluations, mental health check-ins, and mood monitoring offer valuable perspectives on how fasting habits affect vitality and psychological health. By assessing physical performance in both fed and fasted states, the timing of nutrients can be adjusted to maximize exercise benefits. Keeping track of hydration levels and evaluating sleep quality in connection with fasting habits are two more tools that enhance your self-awareness.

Your individual preferences and routines can be accommodated by tailoring fasting windows, and the process is improved by regular self-evaluation, goal alignment, and expert guidance. Those who embrace adaptability and see the process of intermittent fasting as an ongoing educational opportunity are better equipped to make subtle changes that align with their developing self-awareness and promote a deep connection with their bodies and genuine well-being.

Tailoring Intermittent Fasting to Suit Your Unique Path to Wellness

- Starting an intermittent fast is a call to customize the experience to fit your body's preferences and particular rhythms. This exploration is guided by your body type, metabolism, and genetic predispositions. A harmonious integration of fasting methods into your life is ensured when they are in line with your lifestyle, daily routine, and personal choices. Understanding that people have different metabolic rates highlights how crucial it is to give yourself time to adjust when switching between different fasting techniques. Remember that by experimenting with various fasting windows, you can find the one that best suits your energy levels, hunger signals, and general state of health.

- A key component of customizing your intermittent fasting experience is taking into account the timing and makeup of your meals. The personalized approach is strengthened by modifying the timing of nutrient intake according to your daily activities and meal composition to meet your nutritional objectives. A sustainable and fulfilling experience can be ensured by continuously learning from and adapting to your body's reactions to various fasting methods through observation and reflection.

- You can adjust intermittent fasting techniques to fit not just your physical needs but also your social obligations, career schedule, and long-term environmental objectives. You can modify fasting windows based on your hunger signals and daily energy needs by learning to discern between genuine physical hunger and emotional cues. Methodological flexibility creates an approach that changes to meet your changing needs by striking a balance between structure and adaptability.

- Adapting techniques to your own goals is necessary if you want to match your intermittent fasting journey with particular health objectives. If you have underlying medical conditions, it is imperative that you consult healthcare professionals to make sure the method you have chosen is supportive and safe. Understanding how fasting affects stress levels and emotional health leads to deliberate adjustments to practices to support mental health.

- Taking responsibility for your path is essential in this art of personalization. Accepting the freedom to create a customized fasting regimen for yourself encourages ongoing self-improvement. In addition to maximizing the advantages of intermittent fasting, this continuous process of improvement and adaptation paves the way for a profound and long-lasting experience of wellness.

Navigating Wellness

Experimenting with fasting windows is a great way to learn about your body and what works best for you. To do this, you will need to follow through with the list below.

- Starting an intermittent fast is an exciting and private journey, and mastering the art of experimentation is essential to realizing its full potential. Consider beginning with well-known fasting windows such as the 16/8 method or the 14/10 method, and set aside some time for observation to better understand your body's reactions.

- Throughout the fasting window, pay close attention to your body's signals of hunger and energy levels. If the first window of fasting is comfortable, then gradually increase it. Give your body time to adjust to longer periods of time before adjusting further. Try varying the fasting windows on a daily and weekend basis. You can also investigate the effects of changing the timing of meals on satiety and energy.

- It is critical to strike a balance between structure and adaptability. Schedules should be followed consistently, but you should also allow for social gatherings and unforeseen changes in plans. Examine how fasting affects social, professional, emotional, and cognitive facets of life. Keep a fasting journal to record your experiences, noting both the successes and setbacks you encountered while experimenting.

- Consult a dietitian or other medical professional before extending a fast, and make sure to get regular check-ups. Acknowledge your flexibility as a strength and be willing to make small adjustments to your plan when necessary. Think of your exploration as a path toward developing your own expertise in intermittent fasting, and accept the continuous changes that occur in your fasting approach. Recall that the allure of intermittent fasting is its flexibility; through audacious experimentation, you take the first steps toward a life-changing path that is entirely your own.

In conclusion, the synergy between your personal journey and professional guidance forms the cornerstone of a flourishing intermittent fasting experience. As you fine-tune your practices with the wisdom and expertise of healthcare providers and dietitians, you not only optimize your well-being but also cultivate a sustainable and health-driven approach to intermittent fasting.

*****

Having laid the groundwork for a successful intermittent fasting journey, the next chapter delves into the heart of nourishment—optimizing nutrition during eating windows. Uncover the art of crafting meals that not only satisfy your palate but also contribute to your overall health and vitality. Let's embark on a culinary exploration that complements the rhythms of intermittent fasting, ensuring that each bite nourishes your body and fuels your well-being.

Chapter 4:

Optimizing Nutrition During

Eating Windows

When you examine the complex relationship between eating and fasting intermittently, consider every meal as a chance to give your body the fundamental components for thriving health as well as to sate your palate.

Now, we get to go on a gastronomic journey that goes beyond simple nourishment. We explore the skill of choosing nutrient-dense foods, incorporating whole foods for holistic well-being, balancing macronutrients for sustained energy, and avoiding common pitfalls that could impede your nutritional success.

Similar to the rhythmic cycle of intermittent fasting, your eating windows serve as a blank canvas to be painted with vibrant and nutrient-rich colors. Together, we will peel back the layers of culinary lore to find out how to maximize each bite for a happier, healthier you. Remember that every chapter you go through will take you one step closer to achieving a harmonious relationship with food that is in line with your intermittent fasting objectives. This is especially true when we go through the chapters on nutrient-rich choices, macronutrient balance, the attraction of whole foods, and the mindful avoidance of pitfalls.

Are you ready to savor the flavors of nutritional wisdom? Let's dive into the first section and explore the importance of choosing foods that not only tantalize your taste buds but also nourish your body at its core.

Nutrient-Dense Foods

The Importance of Nutrient-Dense Foods

When it comes to the world of nutrition, the spotlight gleams on nutrient-dense foods that serve as powerful allies in your pursuit of optimal health. Picture your plate as a canvas, with each nutrient-rich choice adding depth and vitality to the masterpiece of your well-being. Nutrient-dense foods, packed with vitamins and minerals, go beyond mere calories, fueling cellular processes and supporting overall health. This holistic nourishment not only reduces the risk of chronic diseases but also sustains your energy levels. As you embrace intermittent fasting, each nutrient-rich choice becomes a crucial step toward genuine well-being. So yes, right now, your plate is a canvas. You must allow your choices to craft a masterpiece.

Let's delve into the next movement of our nutritional symphony—balancing macronutrients for a harmonious and energetic composition.

Micro- and Macronutrient Balance in the Ballet of Essential Elements

In the captivating ballet of nutrition, micro- and macronutrients take the stage, choreographing the intricate movements that support your body's functions.

Enough about food; let's make this different and in a fun way. Let's picture the micronutrients as the *petites danseuses*, which encompass essential vitamins and minerals vital for functions ranging from bone health to immune support. The grand performers—proteins, fats, and carbohydrates—are the macronutrients that provide energy for your daily activities. Proteins act as prima ballerinas, supporting muscle maintenance and repair, while healthy fats perform a *pas de deux*, aiding cognitive function and hormonal balance. Carbohydrates will waltz in, supplying energy for tasks, brain function, and exercise. A well-balanced nutrient profile ensures sustained energy release, supporting vitality throughout fasting and feasting periods. Micronutrients play unsung roles in immune function and energy conversion, while macronutrients contribute to essential molecule synthesis.

Imagine your meals as a performance, with each nutrient playing a unique role in the grand spectacle of your health. This probably gives you an idea of how important whatever we put into our mouths actually is. Moving on, let's seamlessly transition into the next movement of our culinary odyssey—exploring the allure of incorporating whole foods into your dietary repertoire.

Balancing Macronutrients

Protein Power, the Backbone of Well-Being

Proteins serve as architects for muscle structure, crucial for maintenance, repair, and overall growth. Beyond muscles, proteins contribute to enzyme, hormone, and immune system component formation, supporting comprehensive health. Partake in diverse protein sources, including plant-based options like legumes, nuts, seeds, and tofu.

Healthy Fats for Satiety to Nourish Mind and Body

Healthy fats promote a sense of fullness after meals, with their unique structure slowing down digestion for prolonged satiety. They play a vital role in supporting cognitive function, especially the omega-3 fatty acids found in chia seeds. Avocado, rich in monounsaturated fats, adds both creaminess and nutritional value.

Carbohydrates for Energy

Carbohydrates are the body's primary energy source for daily activities and fuel for the brain, supporting cognitive function. Always opt for whole grains like quinoa and brown rice, which provide complex carbohydrates for sustained energy release. Always explore a vibrant palette of fruits and vegetables for wholesome carbohydrate options rich in fiber and essential nutrients.

Balancing proteins, healthy fats, and carbohydrates creates a harmonious nutritional symphony, ensuring well-rounded nourishment for your body and mind. Now, let's seamlessly transition into the celebration of incorporating whole foods into your culinary repertoire.

Incorporating Whole Foods

The Whole Food Advantage and Cultivating Optimal Nutrition

Whole, unprocessed foods stand as nutrient powerhouses, offering concentrated vitamins, minerals, and antioxidants. Their minimal processing preserves nutritional integrity, ensuring a full spectrum of health benefits. Embrace the impact of whole foods on gut health, fostering a thriving microbiome and contributing to holistic well-being.

- Choose whole grains like quinoa over refined grains for a nutrient-dense option.

- Opt for fresh fruits instead of canned ones to retain maximum vitamins and antioxidants.

- Include a variety of colorful vegetables in your meals to ensure a broad spectrum of nutrients.

- Incorporate fiber-rich foods like legumes to promote a thriving gut microbiome.

- Let vegetables, whole grains, and lean proteins be the core of your meals, minimizing processed additions.

The Colorful Plate Strategy to Paint Your Plate With Vitality

Implement the colorful plate approach by incorporating a variety of colorful fruits and vegetables, each providing a unique set of nutrients. Showcase the visual appeal and health benefits of a vibrant plate resembling nature's hues. Explore the phytonutrients in plant-based foods, celebrating the joy of a plant-centric diet where whole grains, fruits, and vegetables take center stage.

- Add red tomatoes, green spinach, yellow peppers, and purple eggplant to your plate for diversity.

- Make vegetables and fruits the central focus, relegating processed foods to side roles.

- Include berries for their rich antioxidants or kale for its phytonutrient content.

- Arrange your plate with an artistic flair, making it visually appealing and appetizing.

- Rotate vegetables weekly to expose yourself to different nutrients and flavors.

Envision whole foods as maestros orchestrating a harmonious melody of flavor, nutrition, and visual delight in your meals.

Now, we seamlessly transition into our final movement—navigating common pitfalls that may pose challenges on your intermittent fasting journey.

Abiding Common Pitfalls

Mindful Eating Practices to Stop Overeating

Embrace mindful eating to prevent overconsumption during eating windows. Cultivate a deeper connection with your body's hunger and fullness cues for a balanced and satisfying nutritional experience. So, chew your food slowly, savoring each bite, and put your fork down between bites to avoid overeating. Pay attention to hunger and fullness cues; stop eating when you're satisfied, not overly full.

Hydration Strategies to Ensure Overall Well-Being

Explore the role of hydration in supporting digestion and nutrient absorption. Instill practical strategies for mindful hydration, which we have already looked at, to enhance the nutritional benefits of your meals. Drink water in small amounts every so often, and indulge in herbal teas. Also, drink water throughout the day, especially before meals, to support digestion and prevent overeating.

Navigating Processed Foods and Making Informed Culinary Choices

Delve into the potential drawbacks of processed foods, including hidden sugars and additives, and their impact on health. Equip yourself to read labels with insight and strike a balance between convenience and nutrition with minimally processed, nutrient-rich alternatives.

Always educate yourself first about what will happen when you make a certain decision that will affect your health. Then, navigate the culinary landscape with knowledge and mindfulness, gracefully maneuvering around potential pitfalls. Choose convenience foods consciously, opting for those with minimal processing and high nutritional value.

*****

As we conclude our exploration of optimal nutrition during eating windows, envision your culinary journey as a harmonious symphony— a masterpiece of well-being crafted through nutrient-dense foods, balanced macronutrients, whole foods, and mindful choices. As we get ready to move on to the next chapter, let's consider it the encore to your nutritional symphony. Monitoring and adjusting will fine-tune your intermittent fasting journey, ensuring it remains a dynamic and personalized pursuit of well-being. Join us in the next movement to delve into tracking your journey, recognizing milestones, and making nuanced adjustments for a vibrant, health-infused life. The encore awaits—let's step into the rhythm of progress and adaptation.

Chapter 5:

Navigating the Rhythm of

Transformation

Embarking on the next chapter of your intermittent fasting journey is like stepping into a finely tuned rhythm. What kind of rhythm? Well, it's one that encapsulates progress, awareness, and the art of adaptation. In this chapter, we are going to explore the delicate task of monitoring your journey, recognizing subtle shifts, and making thoughtful adjustments to ensure your path to well-being remains in perfect harmony. Imagine this step as a conductor's baton that is guiding you through the intricate movements of transformation. From tracking changes in weight and body composition to assessing the vitality of your energy and mental clarity, we will be diving deep into the nuanced indicators that paint a vivid portrait of your well-being.

It goes beyond the numerical values on the scale. It's the kind of time where we'll celebrate the victories that go beyond your mass but also how you feel, the energy that propels you, and the mental clarity that sharpens your focus. Let's get ready to shift from quantifiable metrics to qualitative measures that underscore the transformative impact of intermittent fasting. And in the spirit of customization, we'll explore the concept of fine-tuning your fasting schedule to suit your individual needs.

Tracking Changes in Weight and Body Composition

In addition to being a popular weight-loss method, intermittent fasting is becoming more and more of a lifestyle choice with possible health advantages. It's time to learn how to track changes in body composition and weight through intermittent fasting, as well as discover possible obstacles and useful tools or methods for the best outcomes.

How to Put Intermittent Fasting Into Practice

1. First, decide on a fasting protocol.

    o   The 16/8 Method calls for a 16-hour fast window every day, followed by an 8-hour eating window.

    o   The 5:2 diet calls for eating regularly for five days and limiting calories to 500–600 calories on two non-consecutive days.

    o   The eat-stop-eat diet calls for one or two 24-hour fasts per week.

    o   Alternate-day fasting: swapping out days when you eat normally for days when you either fast or eat very little.

2. Try the slow onset.

    o   Initiate your fasting gradually, particularly if it is your first time. As your body adjusts, start with shorter fasting intervals and increase them gradually.

3. Keep yourself hydrated.

   o Staying hydrated is essential when fasting. To stay hydrated without breaking your fast, consider making herbal teas and drinking water on a regular basis.

4. Eat foods high in nutrients.

   o To promote general health, give preference to nutrient-dense foods when breaking your fast. Achieve a balance between healthy fats, carbohydrates, and proteins.

Solving Problems

Now, for the obstacles you could experience and how to solve them:

First Pangs of Hunger

When you are fasting, keep yourself occupied, drink plenty of water, and give your body some time to get used to the new eating schedule.

Always take slow sips of water whenever you feel uncontrollable hunger.

Social Difficulties

Arrange social events around your mealtime or let your loved ones know when you will be fasting.

Variations in Energy

For sustained energy, make sure you are eating meals that are high in nutrients during the designated eating windows.

Overindulging in Food During Meal Times

Recognize your hunger cues, eat mindfully, and refrain from overeating during times when you fast.

Instruments and Methods for Efficient Monitoring

Using Apps for Fasting

Apps like MyFast and Zero can track your fasting windows, track your progress, and give you insights into your fasting experience (Miss, 2020).

Food Journals

Meal-tracking apps like MyFitnessPal or the conventional pen-and-paper journal can help you keep track of your meals and maintain a balanced diet (Wikipedia Contributors, 2019).

Analysis of Body Composition

You can track changes in your body's overall composition, muscle mass, and body fat percentage with devices like DEXA scans or smart scales (CDC, 2021).

Frequent Medical Exams

Well, when it comes to frequent medical check-ups, they will help you guarantee that intermittent fasting is in line with your specific health requirements.

Choosing an appropriate option, dealing with the obstacles, and coming up with efficient tracking tools are all necessary steps in putting intermittent fasting into practice. It can become a sustainable and healthy way of life with the correct resources and some small adjustments along the way. Keep in mind that, yes, the journey may have some initial challenges, so for individualized advice on your intermittent fasting journey, seek the advice of healthcare professionals, stay consistent with routines as well as check-ups, and pay attention to your body.

Evaluating Mental Clearness and Energy With Periodic Fasting

When you start intermittent fasting, it is critical to assess your energy and mental clarity in order to comprehend how this lifestyle affects your overall health. Let's get into how to examine and evaluate these factors, possible difficulties encountered, and methods to maximize energy and cognitive function.

Evaluating Energy Levels

Pay Attention to Your Body

- Throughout the day, keep an eye on your energy levels, particularly when you are fasting or eating.

- Take note of any changes or trends in your energy levels, such as slumps in the middle of the afternoon or increased alertness.

Record Your Everyday Energy Trends

- Maintain a journal to track your energy levels, noting when you are most energized and when you feel tired.

- Log factors, like meal composition, hydration, and sleep quality, that may affect energy levels.

Employ Wearable Technology

- Fitness trackers and other wearables can give you information about your heart rate, amount of physical activity, and sleep quality, in addition to providing a comprehensive look at your energy use.

Evaluate Your Physical Performance

Keep an eye on your performance during exercises or physical activities and record any changes in your strength, endurance, or general stamina. This can help you determine whether or not a particular diet is suitable for your body.

Now, let's discuss some of the challenges that you might face, but we can also look at easy ways for you to overcome these problems.

First Weariness

Give your body time to adjust to the sporadic fasting. To fight fatigue, you can gradually increase the length of your fasts and make sure you are drinking enough water.

Timing of Nutrients

Inappropriate timing of nutrient intake during eating windows can affect energy levels. To maintain energy, try concentrating on nutrient-dense meals that include a balance of proteins, healthy fats, and carbohydrates.

Lack of Water

Dehydration can result from consuming insufficient amounts of water when fasting. Drinking water or herbal teas on a regular basis can help you stay hydrated and boost your energy levels.

Over-Training

Excessive exercise combined with improper rest can make you feel tired. It is important to maintain a well-rounded workout regimen that includes enough downtime to allow your body to heal and avoid burnout.

Evaluating Your Mental Acuity

Coming to the mental part of the journey and making sure that you are not experiencing cognitive decline:

- Take part in mindfulness exercises like deep breathing or meditation.

- Watch how you focus and stay in the moment during these exercises.

- Evaluate your cognitive performance on daily tasks or at work, observing any shifts in your ability to concentrate, be creative, or solve problems.

- Cognitive responsiveness can be measured by timing your response to stimuli, such as visual or auditory cues.

- Assess the quality of your sleep because inadequate or disturbed sleep can seriously impair mental clarity.

Techniques to Improve Cognitive Function

- Plan your meals to fall during periods of high cognitive demand to ensure a steady supply of nutrients to support brain function.

- Include foods that are rich in vitamins, antioxidants, and omega-3 fatty acids, as these are known to support mental wellness (*Foods Linked to Better Brainpower*, 2017).

- Regularly consume large amounts of water as dehydration can impair brain function. Drink water or herbal tea mindfully throughout the day.

- Adopt practices that are adaptogenic to help your body gradually adjust to periods of fasting and build cognitive resilience.

In summary, evaluating mental clarity and energy during intermittent fasting requires a combination of strategic practices, documentation, and self-awareness. Through comprehension of personal patterns, resolution of obstacles, and application of optimization techniques, you can effectively navigate your intermittent fasting journey while maintaining focus on long-term energy and mental health.

Adapting the Intermittent Fasting Schedule to Your Needs

A key to maximizing the advantages of intermittent fasting for specific needs is fine-tuning the fasting schedule. During this process, the fasting windows, meal timing, and duration are adjusted to suit your individual preferences, lifestyle objectives, and health requirements. Let's examine how to adjust a fasting schedule and take individualization into account.

How to Adjust Your Fasting Schedule

To gain insight into your individual preferences, daily schedules, and fluctuations in energy levels throughout the day, conduct a self-evaluation.

- Determine the best times to focus mentally and when hunger is easiest to control.

- Try varying the fasting windows gradually; try 16/8, 18/6, or 24-hour fasts.

- Consider how your body reacts to varying fasting durations and select a window based on personal comfort.

- Sync fasting windows with your body's natural circadian rhythms, taking into account the sleep-wake cycle and the body's peak metabolic hours. Because it synchronizes with the body's internal clock, this alignment can increase the effectiveness of intermittent fasting.

- Consider the timing of your workouts and how they fit into your fasting schedule.

- Try exercising within eating windows or during fasting periods to see which is the best schedule for your own energy needs and level of performance.

- Adjust meal times to suit your lifestyle and tastes. If you have a preference for breakfast, you might select an earlier eating window, whereas another might choose a later one.

- To optimize the nutritional benefits, think about including nutrient-dense meals during certain eating windows.

Aspects to Take Into Account for Individualization

Health Goals

Whether your objectives are to improve metabolic health, gain muscle mass, or control weight, make sure the fasting schedule is in line with those objectives. To make sure that the chosen fasting strategy supports specific health goals, work together with your medical professionals.

Social and Professional Commitments at Work

Adjust the fasting schedule to fit in with your social and professional obligations. In order to improve adherence and sustainability, make sure the fasting window you have selected fits in seamlessly with your regular schedule.

Hunger Cues

Keep an eye out for signs of hunger and modify the fasting schedule as necessary. Finding the right balance between breaking the fast when true hunger strikes and fasting for the length of time necessary to reap the benefits is known as fine-tuning.

Periodic Evaluation

Reevaluate your fasting plan on a regular basis to account for modifications in goals, preferences, or lifestyle. Flexibility is essential to make sure that the fasting strategy can still be adjusted to changing personal needs.

Conscious Compliance

Adopt a mindful approach to following the fasting schedule, keeping in mind your general state of health and comfort. If a fast does not suit your preferences or is causing you undue stress, do not follow it strictly.

The bottom line is that when it comes to intermittent fasting, fine-tuning the fasting schedule requires a customized strategy that takes your lifestyle, health objectives, and personal preferences into account. You can design a fasting schedule that best serves your well-being and encourages sustained adherence to the intermittent fasting lifestyle by following these guidelines and staying aware of your own needs.

*****

To sum up, this customized strategy guarantees the maximum possible benefits of intermittent fasting while simultaneously encouraging long-term commitment to this revolutionary way of living. You know how to assess your body and mind to make sure you are doing what is best for you.

Now, with a focus on weight loss specifically, the next chapter calls for us to get ready as we navigate the finer points of customizing fasting schedules. Expanding on the basis of customized fasting, we will explore the methods, obstacles, and achievements related to utilizing intermittent fasting as a means of achieving efficient and long-term weight loss. Let's move forward and see just how fasting for weight loss can be a transformative experience where mindful practices and purposeful choices come together to create a path toward holistic well-being.

Chapter 6:

Fasting for Weight Loss

Starting a weight loss journey is about more than just losing weight; it is about making a healthy relationship with our bodies. With its cyclical eating and fasting schedule, intermittent fasting offers a dynamic method for reaching and keeping a healthy weight. In this chapter, we will examine the complex mechanisms by which intermittent fasting promotes weight loss, as well as tactics for optimizing fat loss and the benefits of combining exercise and fasting for that all-encompassing weight control.

How Intermittent Fasting Facilitates Weight Loss

Fasting doesn't only limit your food intake at specific times; it goes beyond this. Let's examine *how* closely.

Metabolic Rewiring

Metabolic processes play a key role in the weight loss symphony. A change in how your body uses its energy is orchestrated by intermittent fasting, which functions as a conductor. We can access the complexities of metabolic rewiring—the process by which the body switches from using glucose as its main energy source to effectively burning fat—by welcoming times when we do not eat. This metabolic flexibility becomes an effective tool in the fight against excess weight because fat stores become an easily accessible source of long-term energy.

Hormonal Balancing

Imagine the choreography of hormone balance dictating your body's reactions to food and fasting. When it comes to important hormones, insulin sensitivity is the main focus of intermittent fasting. Insulin levels drop during fasting, which improves your body's capacity to access and use fat stores as fuel. The conductor of fat metabolism and cellular repair, the growth hormone, also steps up, adding to the weight loss process.

Mechanisms of Caloric Deficit

The idea of a caloric deficit—a situation in which your body uses more energy than it takes in—lays the foundation for weight loss. With its set eating windows, intermittent fasting naturally leads to this caloric deficit. The body changes from storing excess calories to burning fat when you adopt controlled energy consumption during the eating window. The end effect is a state of harmonious balance that promotes steady, progressive weight loss.

Now, let's change directions to the finer points of hormonal homeostasis, metabolic rewiring, and the mechanisms of caloric deficit that are orchestrated by periodic fasting. When we dive into the mechanics, try to picture each idea as a unique instrument that adds to the weight loss journey.

Strategies for Maximizing Fat Loss

Starting an intermittent fasting journey for weight loss requires a calculated combination of lifestyle changes, nutrient timing, and mindful eating. Let's go through a few practical methods to optimize fat loss while adhering to an intermittent fasting schedule:

Periods of Strategic Fasting

Customize your fasting periods to maximize your body's ability to burn fat. To use fat that has been stored as energy, think about extending the fasting period. The 16/8 method is a popular strategy that increases fat utilization during the fasting phase by extending the fast to 16 hours.

Calorie-Restrictive Feasting

Though mindful feasting is essential for effective fat loss, intermittent fasting does not prescribe specific calorie limits. During eating windows, choose whole, nutrient-dense foods that emphasize a balance of the nutrients we already looked at: complex carbohydrates, healthy fats, and proteins. This method guarantees that your body gets the nutrients it needs while encouraging a caloric deficit that helps you lose fat.

Integration of Strategic Exercises

Combine intentional exercise programs with fasting periods to enhance fat loss. Along with strength training, you can work out your heart by doing brisk walking or high-intensity interval training. Cardio workouts boost the burning of calories, whereas strength training maintains and increases lean muscle mass, which raises the metabolic rate and improves the efficiency of burning fat (Boutcher, 2011).

Water Content and Thermogenesis

Make the most of water's thermogenic properties and maintain proper hydration when fasting. Water consumption increases metabolism, which helps burn calories. Think about adding herbal teas or cold water; these could boost the thermogenic response and eventually lead to more fat loss.

Include Continual Extended Fasts

Extended fasting on a regular basis, like the 5:2 method or 24-hour fasts, can significantly accelerate fat loss. The body enters a deeper state of ketosis during these longer fasting intervals, where it uses more fat as fuel. These strategies should, however, be used with caution and customized to your tolerance and objectives.

Remember that an all-encompassing strategy that takes into account fasting windows, food selections, exercise regimens, hydration, and occasionally prolonged fasting is the key to optimizing fat loss with intermittent fasting. So, try out these tactics, pay attention to your body, and make the necessary adjustments to find a viable and efficient way to lose fat within the framework of intermittent fasting.

Smart Food Choices

The choices we make when attempting to lose weight during eating windows shape our overall wellness journey. It's time to look into how to choose foods wisely so that you can increase your fat metabolism and achieve sustainable, long-term weight loss.

Methodical Decisions Regarding Fat Metabolism

Making informed food choices that support your weight-loss objectives is more important than deprivation. Think about adding these actions to your repertoire of culinary skills:

- Increase your consumption of protein by consuming foods like tofu and legumes. In addition to helping to maintain muscle mass, protein makes you feel full, which reduces overindulgence in calories.

- Acknowledge the role that healthy fats—found in nuts, seeds, avocados, and olive oil—play in boosting satiety and enhancing brain function. These fats become allies in the pursuit of sustainable weight loss.

- Try complex carbohydrates, opting for whole grains, sweet potatoes, and legumes. These choices provide sustained energy, preventing the erratic blood sugar spikes that can sabotage weight loss efforts.

- Infuse your meals with fiber from fruits, vegetables, and whole grains. Fiber not only promotes digestive health but also contributes to a feeling of fullness, assisting in portion control.

Combining Fasting With Exercise for Weight Management

The combination of exercise and intermittent fasting is a powerful ally in the dynamic interplay of weight management, providing synergistic effects that go beyond calorie burn.

Selecting the Right Exercise Methods

A careful choice of exercise modalities is necessary when starting a weight-management journey that combines exercise and intermittent fasting. Let's step into a short guide for you, showing you how to select suitable exercises that complement your fasting schedule. Let's explore the factors and actions that will enable you to choose exercise modalities that suit your preferences and goals.

Things to Take Into Account When Choosing an Exercise Modality

- Examine the range of exercise modalities in terms of intensity, from low to high.

- When selecting exercises, take into account your current level of fitness, general health, and fasting schedule. Low- to moderate-intensity exercises may be suitable during fasting periods, but high-intensity workouts should be reserved for eating windows.

- Analyze the duration and frequency of your training sessions. Evaluate your commitment to regular physical activity and your availability of time. You may choose to do shorter, more frequent workouts or longer sessions that are timed to coincide with certain eating windows, depending on your fasting schedule.

- Accept workouts that fit your lifestyle and personal preferences. Choosing exercises you enjoy increases the likelihood of sticking to your weight management plan, whether it be at home, in the gym, or outdoors.

How to Select the Right Exercise Modalities

- Start by determining your current level of fitness. If you have never exercised before, you might want to start out with low- to moderate-intensity activities and work your way up as your fitness increases.

- Evaluate the timing of your fasting windows in relation to exercise. Low to moderate-intensity exercises, such as walking or yoga, may be well-suited during fasting periods, providing energy without excessive strain.

- Incorporate diversity into your workout regimen to target various muscle groups and avoid boredom. This might involve a combination of strength training, flexibility training, and cardiovascular exercises.

- Exercise with awareness by paying attention to your body's cues. During times of fasting, if you feel uncomfortable, tired, or lightheaded, reduce the intensity or go for softer activities.

You will empower yourself to choose the exercise modalities that work well with your intermittent fasting journey by carefully weighing the factors and actions listed below. This customized approach guarantees that the exercises you select will enhance your overall well-being and enjoyment of your transformative fitness journey, in addition to helping you manage your weight.

Let's examine a few exercises, but before beginning any new fitness regimen, always remember to speak with a healthcare provider.

Jumping Jacks as a Warm-Up Exercise

- Place your arms at your sides and your feet together as you stand.

- Stretch your arms above your head and jump with your feet wide apart.

- Return to the starting position by jumping.

- Repeat for one to two minutes to raise your body temperature and heart rate.

16/8 Method Exercise With Walking briskly

- Look for a clear, safe place to stroll.

- Start out slowly and go for two to three minutes.

- For the next ten to fifteen minutes, pick up the pace to a brisk walk.

- Allow two minutes for a gentle cool-down to conclude.

Exercise for the 5:2 Diet With High-Intensity Interval Training (HIIT)

- Select a cardiovascular workout (jumping jacks, cycling, running).

- Put in 30 seconds of vigorous work, then take a 30-second break.

- Continue for fifteen to twenty minutes in this fashion.

- Adapt the intensity to your level of fitness.

Eat-Stop-Eat Workout With Resistance Training

- Include weightlifting or bodyweight exercises.

- Try some dumbbell exercises, push-ups, lunges, and squats.

- For each exercise, aim for three sets of ten to twelve repetitions.

- Space out your strength training sessions by 48 hours.

Exercise During an Alternate Day Fast With Cycling or Running

- Depending on your mood, go cycling or running.

- Exercise at a moderate to high intensity when you are not fasting.

- Start out with 20–30 minutes, then extend it over time.

- Pay attention to your body's energy levels and stay hydrated.

Stretching Exercises as a Cool-down

- Give your major muscle groups static stretches.

- Take a few minutes to hold each stretch.

- Stretches for the back, neck, arms, and legs should be included.

- To encourage relaxation during the cool-down, concentrate on deep breathing.

Always adjust the length and intensity of your workouts according to your fitness level and any health issues. Maintaining a regular schedule and making incremental progress will help your workout regimen work better when combined with intermittent fasting.

As we come to the end of our investigation into the benefits of exercise and intermittent fasting for managing weight, picture a harmonious dance between these two effective strategies. A symbiotic relationship that helps you achieve your weight loss goals is built on the thoughtful selection of suitable exercise modalities, well-planned post-fasting activities, and an attentive attitude. Accept this unique journey and realize that combining exercise and fasting is a dynamic, life-changing way of living rather than merely a way to achieve a goal.

*****

Let's now shift our attention to a crucial area of health and well-being: the relationship between diabetes control and fasting. It's time to discover the subtle tactics, factors, and empowering revelations that establish intermittent fasting as a useful ally in the all-encompassing treatment of diabetes. Come explore the possibilities for better glucose regulation, increased insulin sensitivity, and a comprehensive approach to purposeful, intentional diabetes management as we explore the terrain where fasting and diabetes collide.

Chapter 7:

Fasting for Diabetes Management

Starting an intermittent fast is a powerful decision to take control of your blood sugar dynamics and goes beyond simply committing to your health. In this chapter, we will explore the complex relationship between diabetes management and fasting, revealing the significant effects of sporadic fasting on blood sugar regulation. From unraveling the science behind insulin sensitivity to exploring real-life stories of those who have triumphed in diabetes care through fasting, this chapter serves as a guide for a transformative and empowered approach to blood sugar mastery.

As we explore the domains of research and useful advice, get ready to acquire important knowledge that transcends traditional diabetes care. Let's examine how intermittent fasting, which offers a holistic lifestyle shift toward improved health and vitality in addition to a regimen, can be a ray of hope as you navigate the complex terrain of diabetes.

Understanding the Link Between Fasting and Blood Sugar

In order to understand this connection, let's first examine how the body regulates blood sugar.

Food, particularly carbs, is broken down by the body into glucose, which is the main energy source for our cells. The pancreas secretes the hormone insulin, which helps cells absorb glucose and maintain steady blood sugar levels (*Controlling Blood Sugar*, n.d.).

With fasting, the body experiences a metabolic shift. When there is no recent food consumed, the body uses its stored glucose as energy when insulin levels drop. The post-absorptive state, which is this stage, usually starts 8–12 hours after the last meal. This post-absorptive state is prolonged by intermittent fasting, giving the body more time to use its glucose reserves. Consequently, blood sugar levels may drop, particularly if paired with a diet low in carbohydrates and refined sugars. There are various ways in which this drop in blood sugar levels can improve general health.

The Benefits of Fasting on Blood Sugar Levels

The advantages of intermittent fasting for controlling blood sugar include increased insulin sensitivity. Fasting increases a cell's sensitivity to insulin, which improves the hormone's ability to transport glucose into cells. Improved metabolic health and a decreased risk of type 2 diabetes are linked to increased insulin sensitivity. Additionally, intermittent fasting encourages the use of non-traditional energy sources like fatty acids and ketones, which help stabilize blood sugar levels. A major factor in the beneficial effects of fasting on the body's energy dynamics is this metabolic flexibility.

It is important to remember that if you already have blood sugar problems, like diabetes, you should use caution when attempting intermittent fasting. It is best to speak with your healthcare provider to make sure the fasting regimen suits your individual needs.

Side-Effects of Fasting on Diabetics

Moving on, let's now discuss some possible difficulties with blood sugar that may arise while fasting.

Low blood sugar, or hypoglycemia, is a condition that some people may encounter. This may show up as weakness, agitation, or even lightheadedness. It is important to be aware of these symptoms, and if they manifest, you'll need to modify the fasting regimen or consult a healthcare provider. Furthermore, it is critical to routinely check blood sugar levels, particularly for people who already have health issues or are at risk of developing diabetes. Continuous glucose monitoring can provide valuable insights into how the body responds to fasting and help tailor the approach to individual needs.

In summary, knowing the complex relationship between fasting and blood sugar levels reveals the metabolic shift that takes place inside our bodies. When done with awareness, intermittent fasting can help with overall blood sugar regulation, improved insulin sensitivity, and increased metabolic flexibility. It's true that individual reactions might differ, so it is important to proceed cautiously and seek professional assistance when necessary. Keep this knowledge in mind as we continue to investigate intermittent fasting to make sure that fasting and your quest for overall well-being coexist peacefully.

Research and Case Studies on Fasting and Diabetes

Our investigation into the complex relationship between blood sugar and fasting reveals a world where metabolic health is crucial, particularly for people living with diabetes. The various forms of fasting have garnered attention because of their possible effects on insulin sensitivity and blood sugar regulation. This investigation delves deeply into the intricate relationships between blood sugar levels and fasting behaviors, using knowledge from reliable research studies as a guide. By examining this terrain, we get an insight into the concrete advantages and possible drawbacks of fasting, providing insightful information for practical diabetes management solutions. Now, we set out to disentangle the complex relationship between fasting and blood sugar by examining real-world case studies and applying scientific inquiry. Our goal here is to gain a more nuanced understanding of the ways in which these factors interact with one another in the context of metabolic well-being. Let's get started.

A Study Conducted by Dr. Jason Fung

Dr. Jason Fung carried out an extensive study concentrating on its impact on diabetes control. Participants in the study were type 2 diabetics who followed regimens of intermittent fasting. The results showed that blood sugar levels and insulin sensitivity had significantly improved. The potential of fasting as an adjunctive therapy for diabetes was highlighted in Dr. Fung's study (Scibilia, 2019).

Case Study Examining Levels of HbA1c

An interesting case study looked into the connection between diabetes markers and fasting. Participants in the study included people with type 2 and type 1 diabetes who fasted on occasion. The HbA1c levels decreased, according to the results, suggesting better long-term blood sugar control. According to Woerle et al. (2007), this case study raised the possibility that fasting interventions could be an effective way for people to manage their diabetes.

Clinical Trial

A clinical study was carried out to investigate how fasting-like diets affect diabetes. Participants in the study had prediabetes and were given periodic fasting-like interventions. The results showed improved beta-cell function and a drop in fasting glucose levels. This trial shed light on the potential benefits of fasting-mimicking approaches to preventing and managing diabetes (Wei et al., 2017).

All of these studies add to the increasing amount of data that shows fasting has a beneficial effect on diabetes. As we dig deeper into these studies, it becomes clear that intermittent fasting is a promising approach to enhancing different facets of diabetes care. As we acknowledge the important contributions made by these researchers to the advancement of our knowledge regarding fasting in the context of diabetes, let us continue to apply these insights to our daily lifestyle and eating habits.

Practical Tips for Incorporating Fasting Into Diabetes Management

Moving on, you can now come to the conclusion that embarking on the journey of incorporating fasting into diabetes management requires a nuanced understanding and a personalized approach. Let's dive into a few practical tips aimed at empowering you with the tools needed to seamlessly integrate fasting into your diabetes management routine. Let's explore strategies that cater to individual needs, fostering a harmonious balance between the principles of fasting and the intricacies of diabetes care.

Exploring Personalized Strategies for Fasting in Diabetes Management

It's time for some fun as we get to look into methods or tips that you can incorporate into your fasting journey to suit your unique circumstances and foster successful diabetes management.

Sculpting Awareness of Body Responses

Start by cultivating a keen awareness of how your body responds to various fasting methods. Pay attention to nuanced factors such as fluctuations in energy levels, hunger cues, and overall well-being. This self-awareness becomes the cornerstone upon which you'll craft a personalized fasting protocol that harmonizes with your body's distinct rhythms.

Embarking Gradually Into Fasting

If you're new to the realm of intermittent fasting, a gentle initiation paves the way for a smoother transition. Begin with a more lenient fasting window and progressively extend it based on your comfort and tolerance levels. This phased approach gives your body the time it needs to adapt, minimizing potential discomfort and ensuring a sustainable integration into your routine.

Strategic Selection of Fasting Windows

Delve into the art of selecting fasting windows that seamlessly integrate with your daily routine. Whether opting for the popular 16/8 method or a modified schedule tailored to your lifestyle, strategic choices enhance adherence. By aligning your fasting schedule with the ebb and flow of your daily activities, you can integrate this practice seamlessly into your life.

Nurturing Hydration Practices

With diabetes management through fasting, hydration emerges as a vital aspect. Prioritize the intake of an ample amount of water, especially during fasting periods. Adequate hydration not only supports overall health but also acts as a mitigating factor against potential side effects associated with fasting.

Vigilant Blood Sugar Monitoring

When it comes to fasting and diabetes, vigilant monitoring of blood sugar levels becomes a compass guiding your steps forward in this journey. Regularly assess how changes in your fasting routine influence blood sugar levels. This proactive approach empowers you to make informed adjustments, ensuring that your fasting journey aligns seamlessly with your diabetes management goals.

*****

By offering these practical tips tailored to the intricacies of diabetes management, you're now equipped with the knowledge and tools necessary to navigate the journey of intermittent fasting with confidence, resilience, and a focus on individualized well-being.

In summary, our journey through the intricate connection between fasting and diabetes management has equipped you with personalized strategies and practical tips. Now, as we pivot toward the next chapter, let's leverage this newfound wisdom to explore fasting's impact on diverse health aspects. The tapestry of fasting continues, unveiling its potential in various realms of health and well-being.

Chapter 8:

Fasting for Specific Health

Conditions

In the world of health and wellness, targeted fasting emerges as a powerful thread, weaving through the fabric of holistic well-being. As we continue moving forward, our focus shifts to a nuanced exploration of how fasting can be tailored to address specific health conditions. It's a journey beyond the general benefits of intermittent fasting, unlocking the potential of this practice as a personalized tool for health optimization. So, brace yourself for a holistic approach to well-being, where fasting becomes a tailored ally in the pursuit of a healthier and more vibrant life.

Fasting for Metabolic Health

Intermittent fasting transforms metabolism, acting like an urban planner for metabolic processes. Imagine better insulin sensitivity on well-lit streets that facilitate efficient use of glucose and traffic flow. Reducing insulin resistance through intermittent fasting functions as a tactical planner in this metabolic metropolis.

Lipid profiles are like bustling markets in this city. By acting as a wise merchant, intermittent fasting keeps cholesterol in check. Fasting is a guide that helps the dynamic metabolic orchestra play a healthy symphony. It is not just a restriction.

Explore the vibrant marketplaces and streets of metabolism, where the visionary planner reshaping the city for maximum well-being is intermittent fasting. The goal is to create a metabolic masterpiece that exudes vitality rather than merely adhering to restrictions.

Strategic Fasting for Metabolic Harmony

- Begin your fasting journey by embracing the power of the early morning hours. A strategic fasting option often starts with an overnight fast, allowing your body to tap into its fat stores for energy.

- Ditch the traditional three-square-meals-a-day schedule. Some people may find that a shorter 8-hour eating window is the key, while others may benefit more from a longer 12-hour fast. The goal is to find a rhythm that syncs seamlessly with your metabolic clock, enhancing its efficiency.

- Incorporate nutrient-dense meals during feasting periods to fuel your body with the essential building blocks it craves. Proteins, healthy fats, and complex carbohydrates become the notes in this metabolic composition.

- Allow your body to adapt gradually to extended fasting intervals, fostering resilience and ensuring that metabolic harmony becomes a sustainable and enjoyable part of your health journey.

Fasting and Cardiovascular Health

Intermittent fasting is like a silent guardian of cardiovascular well-being. Let's look into the profound connection between intermittent fasting and heart health.

- Because intermittent fasting lowers blood pressure and lessens cardiac strain, it is beneficial to heart health. Intermittent fasting functions as a conductor, balancing lipid profiles and promoting the proper function of HDL and LDL cholesterol.

- Fasting removes oxidative stress debris and inflammation from the arteries, much like a gentle river current does. As a result, arterial pathways remain clear, facilitating easy blood flow and preserving the integrity of the cardiovascular system.

- Additionally, by lowering inflammatory markers and promoting cardiovascular balance, intermittent fasting acts as a break in the overall harmony of health. This ultimately promotes overall heart health by allowing the heart to beat with a gentler rhythm, free from the discordant notes of inflammation.

Guidelines for Cardiovascular Wellness

- Begin your fasting journey with gradual steps. Introduce shorter fasting intervals, allowing your body to adapt to the rhythm of intermittent fasting. A gentle start ensures a smooth transition into heart-healthy practices.

- During eating intervals, prioritize nutrient-rich foods. Opt for a heart-healthy diet rich in fruits, vegetables, lean proteins, and whole grains. This not only complements the fasting process but also provides essential nutrients for cardiovascular well-being.

- Hydration is a key player in cardiovascular health. Ensure that you stay adequately hydrated, especially during fasting intervals. Water supports your body's natural processes and helps maintain optimal blood viscosity.

- Integrate omega-3 fatty acids into your diet. These healthy fats, found in flaxseeds and walnuts, contribute to cardiovascular health. Consider including them in your meals during eating periods for an extra heart-boosting touch.

- Cultivate mindful eating habits. Pay attention to portion sizes and savor the flavors of your meals. Mindful eating not only enhances the fasting experience but also promotes a healthy relationship with food, which is integral to cardiovascular well-being.

- Pair fasting with a regular exercise routine. Physical activity complements the cardiovascular benefits of fasting, promoting heart health. Aim for a combination of aerobic exercises, strength training, and flexibility exercises to keep your heart in top shape.

- Before embarking on any significant dietary changes, especially if you have pre-existing cardiovascular conditions, consult with your healthcare professionals. They can provide personalized guidance based on your health profile and ensure that fasting aligns with your overall well-being.

Remember, the journey to cardiovascular wellness through fasting is not a sprint but a steady marathon. Each step you take toward heart-healthy fasting is a beat in the rhythm of lasting well-being. Following these guidelines will help your heart get pumping to that healthy rhythm.

Fasting for Cognitive Function

Moving forward, it's time to get into the link between fasting and cognitive function, unveiling the neuro-empowering benefits.

- Through the stimulation of brain-derived neurotrophic factor (BDNF) production, intermittent fasting improves cognitive function. This neurotrophic factor functions as a crescendo in brain function, honing cognitive focus. Furthermore, intermittent fasting boosts neuroplasticity, which allows the brain to remodel, reorganize, and adjust, creating a dynamic cognitive environment that is favorable to memory and learning.

- By acting as a caregiver, fasting may protect the brain from the aging process. Fasting's neuroprotective benefits build a defense system around memory that ensures it will last over time.

- The effects of sporadic fasting on hormone levels and neurotransmitter balance support emotional balance and a happy mood within the cognitive symphony.

- When fasting is observed, autophagy is activated, which leads to a thorough cleaning of brain cells. This purging process keeps the cognitive landscape clear and colorful.

As we unravel the cognitive tapestry woven by intermittent fasting, it becomes evident that this practice is not just a tool for physical well-being but a maestro for the mind. The brain-boosting benefits of fasting include focus, neuroplasticity, memory resilience, mood harmony, and detoxification—an opus that elevates your cognitive experience to new heights.

Crafting a Fasting Routine for Brain Health

Seeing the benefits, let's get into the system that will align your fasting intervals with cognitive demands, opting for shorter fasts during mental peaks.

- Give attention to nutrients that strengthen the brain, such as antioxidants and omega-3 fatty acids, when you eat.

- Incorporate herbal teas to support cognitive function and turn drinking more water into a brain-boosting ritual.

- Adopt an adaptogenic fasting lifestyle to build cognitive resilience and enable a gradual transition to longer periods of time.

- Try adjusting the timing of your meals to align with your circadian cycle and boost your cognitive advantages.

- Incorporate brief periods of cognitive rest with stimulating but non-exhaustive activities.

- For sustained cognitive benefits over the long term, establish a regular and sustainable fasting schedule.

- Before making significant changes, consult your healthcare professionals for personalized guidance aligned with cognitive well-being.

Crafting a fasting routine for brain health involves strategic fasting, nutrient-rich feasts, hydration, adaptogenic practices, meal timing, cognitive breaks, consistency, and professional consultation—a symphony that will lead to elevating cognitive clarity and brilliance.

Fasting and Longevity

Not to get too technical, but let's look at a brief breakdown of how fasting can help you live a healthier life for longer.

- Autophagy, a cellular purification and rejuvenation process, is started by intermittent fasting. Maximizing cellular function promotes both general health and the longevity of individual cells.

- Fasting lowers inflammatory markers by acting as a natural extinguisher. It fosters a state of wellness by making the environment unfriendly to age-related illnesses.

- Fasting improves the resilience and efficiency of the mitochondria. It helps maintain vitality, which is essential to solving the longevity conundrum.

- Fasting has the potential to preserve DNA, affect gene expression, and prevent aging-related mutations. It preserves and promotes longevity by shielding the genetic blueprint.

- It helps keep hormones like growth hormone, insulin, and others in balance.

- By promoting metabolic health, fasting creates the foundation for a longer and healthier life.

- A mild stress response brought on by intermittent fasting activates cellular defense mechanisms.

- It increases the body's ability to live a longer, healthier life by preparing it to face the challenges of aging.

When it comes to longevity, intermittent fasting emerges as a beacon, influencing cellular renewal, inflammation reduction, mitochondrial fitness, DNA protection, hormonal harmony, and stress resistance. It becomes a narrative where fasting is a key protagonist in the pursuit of a vibrant and enduring existence.

*****

As we wrap up our exploration of intermittent fasting, it reveals a tapestry of potential and transformation. From diverse fasting methods to benefits spanning weight loss, improved metabolism, cognitive enhancement, and longevity, intermittent fasting proves a versatile ally in the journey toward well-being. So far, we have come to unveil the secrets of aligning meals, crafting brain-boosting fasting routines, and embracing longevity science. The symphony of intermittent fasting resonates for both body and mind, extending its melody to a longer, healthier life.

Moving forward, our journey evolves into a new rhythm, exploring the dynamic partnership of intermittent fasting and exercise in the next chapter. Here, they form a harmonious duet, enhancing each other's benefits for holistic well-being. Join me in this rhythmic exploration, creating a crescendo of vitality, strength, and enduring health. Let the journey continue, echoing the harmony of health through the simple and yet not-so-simple act of fasting.

Chapter 9:

Combining Intermittent Fasting

With Exercise

Now, let's explore how disciplined intermittent fasting and exercise work together to boost health in a powerful partnership. They create a blend of wellness that goes beyond just existing side by side.

As we unravel the secrets of the partnership, envision a journey where each stride, lift, and stretch becomes an integral part of your fasting narrative. Together, intermittent fasting and exercise form a powerful alliance, enhancing each other's benefits and paving the way for a holistic approach to well-being. Sound fascinating? Well, let's embark, move forward, and look where the fusion of fasting and exercise creates a symphony of vitality, strength, and enduring health.

The Evolution Between Fasting and Exercise

This partnership extends beyond individual health practices, creating a symphony of well-being that resonates through every aspect of your life. At first, it may sound daunting, especially if you think about movement on an empty stomach. But remember that with intermittent fasting, there are only select times when you won't be fully satiated. As we have already seen, you will have the option of selecting the best time for you to exercise depending on your needs.

Metabolic Benefits of Intermittent Fasting and Exercise

The combination of intermittent fasting and exercise enhances metabolic functions. Intermittent fasting optimizes nutrient utilization and prompts a shift from glycogen to fat stores for energy. This process aids in effective weight management and improved metabolic health. Additionally, the preservation of muscle mass is a notable outcome. Exercise stimulates muscle growth, while intermittent fasting mitigates excessive muscle breakdown, ensuring the maintenance and resilience of muscles during fitness pursuits.

Furthermore, this combined approach positively influences insulin sensitivity. Intermittent fasting, paired with exercise, lowers the risk of insulin-related issues and promotes stable blood sugar levels, contributing to overall metabolic well-being. The integration of intermittent fasting and exercise also improves endurance by enhancing the body's ability to efficiently utilize energy stores. This adaptation prepares your body for prolonged physical activity and increases stamina.

In terms of cognitive benefits, the combination fosters cognitive harmony. Intermittent fasting's positive impact on cognitive functions, coupled with exercise's promotion of mental clarity, results in improved focus, memory, and overall cognitive well-being. Collectively, these effects create a metabolic strategy that supports holistic well-being and vitality.

As we examine the benefits of both fasting and exercise, picture every facet of your health aligning with this potent partnership. This holistic approach to health optimization is not just about fitness goals; it's about creating a rhythm of vitality that echoes through every facet of your life. So, one question: Are you ready to join the journey where intermittent fasting and exercise unite, unlocking the door to comprehensive well-being?

Unlocking Common Physiological Pathways

It's the moment of the big reveal, where we uncover the shared mechanisms that bind intermittent fasting and exercise in a symbiotic embrace. Beyond their individual merits, the fusion of these health practices amplifies their impact, creating a combination that resonates through your body's intricate workings.

- Both intermittent fasting and exercise actively stimulate autophagy, enabling cells to eliminate damaged components. This serves as a fundamental mechanism for cellular rejuvenation, contributing significantly to overall health and longevity (Shabkhizan et al., 2023).

- Intermittent fasting and exercise work together to enhance mitochondrial health. Fasting triggers mitochondrial biogenesis, generating new mitochondria, while exercise optimizes their efficiency. This acts as a robust force, fueling the body's energy production and fortifying resilience.

- Fasting and exercise jointly influence hormonal regulation, with insulin, growth hormone, and other key hormones performing in coordination. This not only supports metabolic health but also creates an environment conducive to muscle preservation and fat burning.

- Both intermittent fasting and exercise collaborate to reduce inflammation markers. This creates a harmonious melody of wellness, establishing an environment less favorable to chronic diseases and promoting overall health.

- Individually, both fasting and exercise enhance brain function, and when integrated, their impact forms a powerful symphony. This contributes to improved cognitive function, heightened neuroplasticity, and increased mental clarity.

- Intermittent fasting and exercise synergize to improve insulin sensitivity, a critical factor in blood sugar control. This reduces the risk of insulin-related health issues, ensures stable glucose levels, and supports overall metabolic health.

Choosing the Right Exercise Routine

In the interplay between intermittent fasting and exercise, the right choice of exercise routine becomes a crucial orchestrator of success. Tailoring your exercise to complement specific fasting methods ensures a harmonious partnership that maximizes health gains. Here's guidance on the best exercise modalities that synchronize seamlessly with different fasting options.

16/8 Method: Consistent Cardio Cadence

Incorporate a consistent cardio cadence into the 16/8 method, marked by a daily fasting window. Go for moderate-intensity cardiovascular exercises like brisk walking, jogging, or cycling. These activities facilitate fat-burning during fasting periods, promoting metabolic flexibility.

5:2 Diet: Strategic Strength Training

Complement the intermittent calorie restriction of the 5:2 diet with strategic strength training. Engage in resistance exercises such as weightlifting or bodyweight workouts on non-fasting days. This approach preserves lean muscle mass and boosts metabolism, aligning with the principles of intermittent fasting.

Eat-Stop-Eat: Intermittent Intensity Peaks

Optimize the eat-stop-eat method, featuring 24-hour fasting intervals with intermittent intensity peaks. Incorporate high-intensity interval training (HIIT) during eating periods to enhance fat-burning and metabolic benefits.

These brief, intense exercises align with the rhythm of eat-stop-eat.

Alternate-Day Fasting: Endurance Endeavors

Embrace endurance endeavors to complement the uniqueness of ADF. Include activities like running, swimming, or cycling on non-fasting days to tap into sustained energy stores. This approach supports the fasting rhythm and contributes to overall cardiovascular health.

A Personalized Approach

Move beyond specific fasting methods and adopt a personalized approach to exercise. Pay attention to your body's cues and preferences, whether it's yoga, Pilates, or a dance class. The key is finding joy in movement and aligning your exercise routine with your lifestyle for a sustainable and enjoyable health journey.

Remember, the right exercise routine is not a one-size-fits-all concept. It's a melody that should resonate with your fasting rhythm and individual preferences. By tailoring your exercise to complement specific fasting practices, you create a symphony of wellness that harmonizes with your unique health journey. So don't let fear stop you. Join the exploration, where exercise and fasting become collaborative partners in the pursuit of holistic well-being.

Creating a Holistic Fitness Plan

Crafting a well-rounded exercise routine within the context of intermittent fasting is similar to composing a symphony of health. Here's a blueprint to guide you in creating a holistic fitness plan that harmonizes seamlessly with your fasting journey:

- Clarify your fitness objectives, be they weight loss, muscle building, or overall well-being, to shape your exercise routine.

- Align your workouts with your chosen intermittent fasting method, considering fasting windows for optimal combination between fasting and exercise.

- Blend cardiovascular and strength-training exercises for a balanced approach. Cardio enhances fat burning, while strength training preserves muscle mass and boosts metabolism.

- Incorporate activities like yoga or Pilates for joint health, flexibility, and overall body mobility into your fitness plan.

- Prioritize regular, moderate-intensity workouts over sporadic high-intensity sessions for sustainable fitness aligned with intermittent fasting.

- Tune into your body's signals, adapting workout intensity or timing based on fatigue or hunger for a healthy and sustainable exercise routine.

- Ensure proper hydration, especially during fasting periods. Refuel post-exercise with nutrient-dense meals to support recovery.

- Keep your routine dynamic by diversifying exercises and targeting different muscle groups to prevent monotony and add enjoyment to your fitness plan.

- Consider guidance from fitness professionals, especially if you're new to exercise or intermittent fasting, for personalized advice aligned with your goals.

- Acknowledge all of your achievements, whether completing a challenging workout or reaching a fitness milestone, to reinforce your commitment to a holistic and sustainable health journey.

Now, let's get into the part where eating and exercising come together in the fasting journey.

Pre- and Post-Workout Nutrition

So, what exactly is there to discover on nutrition strategies before and after workouts within the context of intermittent fasting? Understanding how to fuel your body during these crucial periods enhances the symbiotic relationship between exercise and fasting.

Pre-Workout Fueling

- First, plan your pre-workout meal strategically within your fasting window. Consume a balanced meal with a mix of carbohydrates, protein, and healthy fats about 1–2 hours before exercising. This provides sustained energy without compromising the benefits of fasting.

- Prioritize hydration before your workout. Adequate water intake is essential for optimal performance. Consider adding electrolytes to maintain electrolyte balance if you're exercising during a fasting period.

- If you prefer working out in a fasted state, consider a small, easily digestible snack 30–60 minutes before exercising. Options like a banana, a handful of nuts, or a protein smoothie can provide a quick energy boost.

Post-Workout Nourishment

- After your workout, prioritize protein intake to support muscle repair and growth. Include a protein-rich meal or snack within the post-exercise window, ideally within 30 minutes to an hour.

- Replenish glycogen stores with a mix of carbohydrates and protein in your post-workout meal. This combination enhances recovery and prepares your body for the next workout.

- Hydration is crucial post-exercise. Replenish lost fluids by drinking water throughout the day. Consider adding a source of electrolytes for enhanced rehydration, especially if you've engaged in intense or prolonged exercise.

- Pay attention to hunger and energy levels after your workout. If you're hungry, prioritize a nutrient-dense meal to refuel. If you're not hungry, ensure you stay hydrated and listen to your body's cues for nourishment.

Supplements in Moderation

While intermittent fasting emphasizes whole foods, supplements can be considered if needed. Branched-chain amino acids (BCAAs) or protein supplements can support muscle recovery. However, it's essential to maintain a balanced and varied diet. Before incorporating supplements, especially if you have specific health conditions, consult with your healthcare professional or a nutritionist for personalized guidance.

Understanding the nuances of pre- and post-workout nutrition during intermittent fasting empowers you to optimize your exercise routine while maintaining the integrity of your fasting practice. Whether it's strategic fueling before a workout or thoughtful nourishment post-exercise, these fueling strategies enhance the combination of intermittent fasting and exercise for a holistic approach to health and fitness.

Enhancing Performance and Recovery With the Art of Nutrient Timing

There is a key element in unlocking peak exercise performance and fostering optimal recovery within the framework of intermittent fasting. Discover the strategic alignment of nutrients with your fasting rhythm to elevate your fitness journey. Let's look into the art of nutrient timing.

Strategic Pre-Workout Nutrition

- Include complex carbohydrates in your pre-workout meal for sustained energy. Whole grains, fruits, or vegetables can be effective sources.

- Combine carbohydrates with moderate protein for energy and muscle maintenance. Options like a banana with nut butter or yogurt with fruit strike a balanced mix.

- Ensure adequate hydration before exercising to prevent impaired performance. Sip water or electrolyte-rich beverages leading up to your workout.

Intra-Workout Hydration

- Maintain hydration during your workout, especially in prolonged or intense sessions, to support performance and prevent dehydration-related fatigue.

- For longer workouts or when fasting, incorporate electrolytes through beverages or natural sources like coconut water to replenish losses from sweat.

Post-Workout Nutrient Replenishment

- Follow your workout with a protein-rich post-exercise meal to aid muscle repair. Options like plant-based proteins or protein shakes contribute to effective recovery.

- Replenish glycogen stores with a mix of carbohydrates and protein in your post-workout meal, supporting recovery and preparing for the next exercise bout.

- Integrate anti-inflammatory foods like fruits, vegetables, and omega-3-rich foods into your post-workout nutrition to mitigate exercise-induced inflammation and enhance recovery.

Individualized Approach

- Pay attention to how your body responds to nutrient timing. Adjust your approach based on energy levels, hunger cues, and overall well-being.

- Periodically experiment with different nutrient timing strategies, adapting based on your evolving fitness goals and personal preferences.

Professional Guidance

For specific fitness goals or dietary considerations, seek guidance from nutrition and fitness professionals. Their expertise can provide tailored advice aligned with your individual needs.

By mastering the art of nutrient timing within the fasting framework, you amplify the benefits of exercise, optimize performance, and pave the way for efficient recovery. This strategic alignment of nutrients with your fasting rhythm is not just a science; it's an art that propels you toward peak fitness and well-being.

*****

Coming to the end, as one chapter closes, another unfolds. The final segment of our expedition beckons—a chapter that transcends the confines of a dietary strategy and transforms intermittent fasting into a lifestyle. It's not just about fasting for a season but adopting a rhythm that resonates with life itself.

In the coming chapter, we delve into the profound concept of "Fasting for Life." It extends beyond the confines of a mere dietary pattern, embracing fasting as an enduring companion in the journey of life. From sustainable practices to mindful choices, join us in uncovering how intermittent fasting transcends into a lifestyle—a mindful and purposeful way of navigating the tapestry of existence. As we turn the page, anticipate not just the closing chapter but the dawn of a lifestyle enriched by the rhythm of fasting for life.

Chapter 10:

Fasting for Life

From the last leg of our journey—an adventure that knows no bounds to space or time—this chapter serves as more than just a conclusion; it is a call to accept fasting as a constant partner in life's vast scheme. This chapter is not just an epilogue; it's an invitation to embrace fasting as an enduring companion in the grand territories of life.

As we delve into sustainable practices, mindful choices, and the integration of fasting principles into the fabric of everyday existence, prepare to witness the metamorphosis of intermittent fasting. It's no longer a mere strategy; it's a way of life—an approach worth navigating, a purposeful and mindful vast and intricate landscape of our existence.

Making Intermittent Fasting a Sustainable Lifestyle

Cultivating a Lifelong Practice

Let' go beyond the trend by developing intermittent fasting as a lifetime habit that calls for consideration and flexibility.

Consider fasting a more mindful practice that takes into account your body's individual needs and gives you flexibility in your fasting schedule rather than seeing it as a passing fad. Instead of following strict regimens, gradually incorporate fasting and make adjustments in response to your body's needs. This will help you build a foundation of tolerance and flexibility.

In order to keep your routine varied and comprehensive, embrace diversity by investigating different intermittent fasting techniques and switching between them. Adapt your fasting routine to the varying seasons of life while acknowledging your body's changing needs. Make nutrient-dense meals a priority during eating windows to support the fasting rhythm. This will promote general well-being.

Make a deep connection with your body's signals of hunger and fullness, and allow your intuitive eating to inform your dietary decisions.

Share your fasting experience with others to help you navigate social situations with grace. Strike a balance that permits connection without sacrificing your commitment.

To deal with emotional aspects, practice mindfulness and always try to ensure that intermittent fasting has a positive effect on your mental and emotional health.

You must, as is necessary with every aspect of life, celebrate your progress toward achieving specific fasting goals, increased energy, or better general health as you reach new milestones on your intermittent fasting journey.

A lifetime practice of intermittent fasting entails more than just following dietary guidelines; it also entails an ongoing conversation, experimentation with different fasting rhythms, and a seamless integration into your own life's narrative. Think of it not as a short-term event, but rather as a friend who will be with you as you navigate the various stages of your life.

Developing a Fasting Habit

Smooth Incorporation Into Everyday Life

To incorporate intermittent fasting into your daily routine, you must take a deliberate and pleasurable approach. This makes it more easily acceptable and forces your mind to look through a pair of positively tinted spectacles as you take to fasting religiously and diligently.

Do take into account the following pointers to easily develop a habit of fasting that fits in with your life's rhythm:

- Set regular fasting windows aligned with your circadian rhythms and daily activities.

- Sync fasting hours seamlessly with your lifestyle, making it second nature.

- Cultivate surroundings that support your fasting journey, removing unnecessary temptations.

- Designate specific spaces for eating, reinforcing positive eating habits.

- Plan and prepare meals in advance to minimize decision fatigue.

- Keep hydration options readily available, integrating them into your fasting routine.

- Begin fasting windows with intention setting, reflecting on goals and positive impacts.

- Mindfully break your fast, adding a conscious element to the experience.

- Schedule enjoyable activities during fasting hours to infuse joy into the experience.

- Embrace culinary exploration and the pleasure of trying new recipes.

- Acknowledge achievements, celebrate completing longer fasts, or adhere to your schedule.

- Use positive affirmations to reinforce commitment and recognize the benefits.

Cultivating intermittent fasting as a habit is a journey of intention, consistency, and joy. When you incorporate fasting into your everyday routine, it becomes a pleasurable and rhythmic habit that is ingrained in your being.

You will need to let your fasting habit flow naturally with the tune of your life as you set out on this journey.

Incorporating Fasting Into Social Life

We have gone over this previously, but to touch on some added life context, managing social situations while on an intermittent fast entails adjusting your fasting schedule to fit in with get-togethers, shared meals, and experiences. The following useful advice will help you adjust intermittent fasting to your social life:

- Inform friends and family about your intermittent fasting experience and your health objectives in an honest manner.

- When you communicate your fasting schedule and objectives during social gatherings, you set expectations.

- Schedule eating times around group meals and fasting windows around social events.

- Accept adaptability and remain devoted while modifying your fasting schedule for special occasions.

- When eating, choose meals that are high in nutrients, especially when you are with other people.

- Moderation is key to ensuring the enjoyment of indulgences without sacrificing health objectives.

- Prior to social gatherings, plan your fasting strategy, taking goals, timing, and food options into account.

- When faced with situations where food options are limited, carry snacks that are suitable for fasting.

- Engage in social activities with awareness, abstain from eating, and emphasize making connections.

- Celebrate with symbolic actions like toasts as you honor your fasting commitment.

- Encourage social interactions that are not food-related to diversify the activities you propose.

- Create a network of people who are understanding and respectful of your fasting journey and who can support you.

Adapting intermittent fasting to your social life requires thoughtful decision-making, flexibility, and open communication. You can sync your fasting rhythm with the bonds of connections and shared experiences by navigating social situations with intention and balance.

With this journey begun, try to incorporate fasting into your social life so that every get-together offers a chance to make deep connections and receive nourishment.

Sharing Your Fasting Journey

It can be a life-changing experience to share your intermittent fasting journey with loved ones, as it can promote empathy and understanding.

Cultivating Understanding and Support

Here's how to openly and honestly explain your fasting lifestyle to others:

- Learn about the benefits, principles, and alignment of intermittent fasting with your goals.

- Be prepared with concise, well-thought-out responses to concerns in response to anticipated questions.

- Establish a relaxed environment for the talk by steering clear of hectic or stressful times.

- To guarantee receptivity, schedule the conversation for a specific time.

- Discover and write down in a journal your personal reasons for implementing intermittent fasting, such as improving your general health or managing your weight.

- Emphasize your lifestyle and health objectives and how fasting helps you achieve them.

- Define the particular fasting technique you have selected and dispel any misunderstandings.

- Make it clear that intermittent fasting is a planned eating strategy rather than starvation.

- Emphasize the advantages and good experiences you have had since starting intermittent fasting.

- Promote open communication by stimulating curiosity and asking and answering questions.

- Stress that this is a personal journey and extend an invitation to others who might be interested in joining.

- Acknowledge people's freedom of choice while assuring them that your choice does not affect others.

- Thank them for their support and understanding as you wrap up the talk.

- Recognize the value of having a candid conversation about lifestyle decisions.

By sharing your intermittent fasting journey authentically and openly, you create a foundation for understanding and support. Your experience becomes a shared journey, and those around you may gain insights into the positive impact of intermittent fasting on overall well-being.

As you navigate these conversations, allow understanding, compassion, and support to flourish within your social circle with open communication. This will bridge a very large gap.

Nurturing Long-Term Well-Being With Intermittent Fasting

Embarking on a lifelong intermittent fasting journey is a dynamic commitment to sustained well-being. To navigate this transformative path, consider these ongoing health maintenance strategies:

- Make routine examinations a priority in order to keep an eye on important health indicators.

- Have candid discussions regarding your fasting lifestyle with your medical professionals.

- Modify fasting schedules in response to your age, health issues, or changes in lifestyle.

- Pay attention to your body's cues so that you can adjust for a smooth and peaceful fasting experience.

- During meal times, concentrate on eating a well-balanced, nutrient-rich diet.

- For particular nutrient needs, take into consideration supplements based on advice from your medical professionals.

- Make maintaining hydration a priority during your fast.

- When selecting hydration-boosting drinks, keep eating windows in mind.

- Include a fun and long-lasting workout regimen in your daily life.

- Exercise regimens should be adjusted to the evolving physical demands of various life stages.

- Make stress reduction a priority by engaging in mindfulness exercises.

- Stress the importance of restful sleep for general health.

- Make ties with a community of people who are supportive and have health objectives similar to yours.

- Learn about the relationship between intermittent fasting and holistic health practices.

Using holistic health strategies is necessary to navigate a lifetime of intermittent fasting. These include adaptability, prioritizing nutrition, staying hydrated, incorporating physical activity, and fostering community support, helping you establish a foundation for sustained well-being.

With each checkpoint on this path, you are reaffirming your commitment to lifelong health and vitality.

Navigating Fasting Practices Through Life Transitions

Life is a journey filled with transitions and transformations, and mastering the art of adapting intermittent fasting to life's changes ensures your well-being takes precedence.

To flexibly adjust your fasting practices:

- Acknowledge distinct life phases with unique demands.

- Embrace flexibility as a key to sustainable intermittent fasting.

- Adjust fasting routines during busy work or travel periods.

- Prioritize health while balancing work commitments and travel requirements.

- Adapt fasting methods to accommodate parenting responsibilities.

- Explore family-friendly fasting that aligns with shared meal times.

- Be attuned to health shifts with age and adjust fasting practices accordingly.

- Consult your healthcare professionals for personalized guidance during health challenges.

- Modify fasting routines during times of heightened stress or emotional changes.

- Integrate mindfulness practices to enhance your emotional well-being.

- Embrace flexibility on special occasions for an enjoyable experience.

- Approach festive meals mindfully, balancing intermittent fasting with occasional indulgences.

- Revisit personal health goals during life transitions.

- Set realistic expectations and understand that adaptation is a natural part of the intermittent fasting journey.

Adapting to life's changes is intrinsic to the intermittent fasting adventure. By infusing flexibility, mindfulness, and a willingness to evolve, you empower yourself to navigate transitions seamlessly. With every adjustment, it becomes a conscious choice, guided by the compass of well-being, as you gracefully flow through the ever-changing currents of life.

In life, change is the one constant, and adjusting intermittent fasting practices to life's flow becomes a dance of resilience and wellness. Now, you have learned how to navigate transitions while staying committed to your well-being. Flexibility is not a compromise but a tool for sustainability. Life's twists are opportunities for growth. Whether embarking on new adventures, parenting, or aging gracefully, you are allowed to and can definitely tailor your fasting journey to harmonize with every phase. In the songs of change, find the melody of well-being.

Remember, each modification is a conscious choice, a note in the evolving composition of your health journey. Stay connected to your core goals, nurturing both physical and emotional vitality.

Your fasting journey isn't a rigid set of rules but a dynamic expression of commitment to a vibrant life. Embrace flux, dance with transitions, and savor each moment. In this intricate process, let Lao Tzu's wisdom guide you: "Life is a series of natural and spontaneous changes. Don't resist them; that only creates sorrow. Let reality be reality. Let things flow naturally forward in whatever way they like" (n.d.).

May these words inspire grace and resilience as you adapt intermittent fasting to life's ever-changing path.

Conclusion

As we come to the end of the transforming domains of intermittent fasting, it is important that we take a moment to consider the profound knowledge that we have gained along the way. Every chapter has served as a springboard for a comprehensive strategy for health and well-being that goes beyond traditional dietary paradigms.

When we look again at the key takeaways from our shared experience, we see a thread of mental strength, metabolic regeneration, and the elegant integration of fasting into daily life. But as it stands now, think of it as a bridge, a connection between what you have learned and how you can use it in your daily life rather than the end. Instead of following a straight line, intermittent fasting is a dynamic journey marked by constant self-discovery, progress, and occasional setbacks.

Winston Churchill famously said, "It is the courage to continue that counts. Success is not final, and failure is not fatal" (De Win, 2023). This emotion perfectly sums up your experience with intermittent fasting. Enjoy your successes and your advancements; when you encounter challenges, keep in mind that you are strong and that you should press on. Apply this journey's wisdom to your daily decisions, for it is through these that transformation persists over time. You are the author and protagonist of your own happiness; this book is merely meant to serve as a reference.

The resources provided should not be viewed as mere references as you continue to explore the fascinating field of health and wellness; rather, view them as partners in your never-ending quest for knowledge. When the last page is turned, the journey does not end; rather, it begins a new chapter in which you can impact your own well-being.

I wish you well-being, a robust sense of energy, and the self-assurance that results from managing your own health. May you stay motivated and well as your fasting journey unfolds with purpose and intention.

References

Boutcher, S. H. (2011). High-intensity intermittent exercise and fat loss. *Journal of Obesity*, *2011*, 1–10. https://doi.org/10.1155/2011/868305

Building, burning, and storing: how cells use food. (n.d.). Learn Genetics. https://learn.genetics.utah.edu/content/metabolism/bbs

CDC. (2021, December 28). *Radiation in healthcare: Bone density (DEXA Scan) | Radiation*. https://www.cdc.gov/nceh/radiation/dexa-scan.html#:~:text=DEXA%20(dual%20x%2Dray%20absorpti ometry

Controlling blood sugar. (n.d.). Diabetes Education Online. https://dtc.ucsf.edu/types-of-diabetes/type2/understanding-type-2-diabetes/how-the-body-processes-sugar/controlling-blood-sugar/#:~:text=Insulin%20is%20the%20main%20regulator

De Win, J. (2023, July 7). *Success is not final, failure is not fatal: it is the courage to continue that count*. LinkedIn. https://www.linkedin.com/pulse/success-courage-continue-count-john-de-win

Fletcher, J. (2019, May 31). *Why is sleep important? 9 reasons for getting a good night's rest*. Medical News Today. https://www.medicalnewstoday.com/articles/325353

Foods linked to better brainpower. (2017, May 30). Harvard Health. https://www.health.harvard.edu/healthbeat/foods-linked-to-better-brainpower#:~:text=Leafy%20greens%20such%20as%20kale

Franklin, B. (n.d.). *Benjamin Franklin quotes.* Goodreads. https://www.goodreads.com/quotes/8792993-the-best-of-all-medicines-are-resting-and-fasting

Gunnars, K. (2021, May 13). *10 evidence-based health benefits of intermittent fasting.* Healthline. https://www.healthline.com/nutrition/10-health-benefits-of-intermittent-fasting

Gupta, S. (2023, March 22). *This type of fasting isn't safe long term: Here's what to do instead.* Mindbodygreen. https://www.mindbodygreen.com/articles/alternate-day-fasting#:~:text=Science%2Dbacked%20benefits%20of%20alternate

Intermittent fasting: What is it, and how does it work? (2023, September 29). Hopkinsmedicine. https://www.hopkinsmedicine.org/health/wellness-and-prevention/intermittent-fasting-what-is-it-and-how-does-it-work#:~:text=Young%20men%20who%20fasted%20for

Miss, D. (2020, November 2). *How the Zero app can help with intermittent fasting.* Medium. https://lorichappellmann.medium.com/how-the-zero-app-can-help-with-intermittent-fasting-19eaf2d8551d

Naous, E., Achkar, A., & Mitri, J. (2023). Intermittent fasting and its effects on weight, glycemia, lipids, and blood pressure: A narrative review. *Nutrients, 15*(16), 3661. https://doi.org/10.3390/nu15163661

Nencioni, A., Caffa, I., Cortellino, S., & Longo, V. D. (2018). Fasting and cancer: molecular mechanisms and clinical application. *Nature Reviews. Cancer, 18*(11), 707–719. https://doi.org/10.1038/s41568-018-0061-0

Schübel, R., Graf, M. E., Nattenmüller, J., Nabers, D., Sookthai, D., Gruner, L. F., Johnson, T., Schlett, C. L., von Stackelberg, O., Kirsten, R., Habermann, N., Kratz, M., Kauczor, H.-U., Ulrich, C. M., Kaaks, R., & Kühn, T. (2016). The effects of intermittent calorie restriction on metabolic health: Rationale and study design of the HELENA Trial. *Contemporary Clinical Trials*, *51*, 28–33. https://doi.org/10.1016/j.cct.2016.09.004

Scibilia, R. (2019). The Diabetes Code: Prevent and Reverse Type 2 Diabetes Naturally. *Clinical Diabetes*, *37*(3), 302–303. https://doi.org/10.2337/cd19-0025

Shields, D. A. (2020, December 12). *A comprehensive guide to fasting: Timeline, stages & benefits.* Dr. Alexis Shields. https://dralexisshields.com/guide-to-fasting

Tzu, L. (n.d.). *Lao Tzu quotes.* BrainyQuote. https://www.brainyquote.com/quotes/lao_tzu_151126

Vasim, I., Majeed, C. N., & DeBoer, M. D. (2022). Intermittent fasting and metabolic health. *Nutrients*, *14*(3), 631. https://doi.org/10.3390/nu14030631

Villines, Z. (2021, January 28). *Fat digestion: How it works and more.* Www.medicalnewstoday.com. https://www.medicalnewstoday.com/articles/fat-digestion#fat-digestion

Wang, Y., & Wu, R. (2022). The effect of fasting on human metabolism and psychological health. *Disease Markers*, *2022*, 1–7. https://doi.org/10.1155/2022/5653739

Wei, M., Brandhorst, S., Shelehchi, M., Mirzaei, H., Cheng, C. W., Budniak, J., Groshen, S., Mack, W. J., Guen, E., Di Biase, S., Cohen, P., Morgan, T. E., Dorff, T., Hong, K., Michalsen, A., Laviano, A., & Longo, V. D. (2017). Fasting-mimicking diet and markers/risk factors for aging, diabetes, cancer, and cardiovascular disease. *Science Translational Medicine*, *9*(377), eaai8700. https://doi.org/10.1126/scitranslmed.aai8700

What is the 5:2 diet? (n.d.). BBC Good Food. https://www.bbcgoodfood.com/howto/guide/what-52-diet

Wikipedia Contributors. (2019, April 24). *MyFitnessPal.* Wikipedia; Wikimedia Foundation. https://en.wikipedia.org/wiki/MyFitnessPal

Woerle, H. J., Neumann, C., Zschau, S., Tenner, S., Irsigler, A., Schirra, J., Gerich, J. E., & Göke, B. (2007). Impact of fasting and postprandial glycemia on overall glycemic control in type 2 diabetes. *Diabetes Research and Clinical Practice*, *77*(2), 280–285. https://doi.org/10.1016/j.diabres.2006.11.011

Printed in Great Britain
by Amazon

40573958R00086